Testimonials

"The book discusses the perceived rise of a global totalitarianism under the cover of the COVID-19 pandemic, framing it as a spiritual and moral crisis that challenges the concept of objective reality and sacred truth. The thesis is persuasive; the argument forceful; the writing colorful; and the diagnosis and cure provocative. Still, all this is not entirely new; indeed, the cure recalls the traditional idea of Catholic and liberal education which revolutionized European culture and progressively the world. For instance, Kozinski particularly stresses the reading of Plato and Shakespeare alongside the Bible. He proposes the founding on such a basis of a new university: RCU or Real Christian University. Such liberal arts education is crucial, he says, but it is not enough. There must also be an existential encounter with God; not with mere doctrine (secular or religious): the whole man, body and soul, must be formed."

— Peter Simpson,
Professor Emeritus of Philosophy and Classics,
City University of New York

"Everything, literally everything, they told us in 2020 and after was a lie, and these lies were aimed at the total subjugation of society and human souls." So writes Thaddeus Kozinski in an uncompromising critique of the spiritual rot engendered by the Western Enlightenment and political liberalism, culminating in an unprecedented attack on human dignity by the governments of liberal democracies during the "Covid-19" debacle. The reason why populations allowed this to happen was their "obedience to the Sacred State and the demonic voice speaking through it." Too many people have turned away from the Good, the True, and the Beauti-

i

ful — from God — and are instead willing to live in a manufactured un-reality. Only a reorientation of the social and political order around the truths revealed in the Catholic tradition and aspiration towards holiness of soul offer any hope of a remedy. Yet, with so many people choosing unreality, not least those hiding beneath a pious facade, and with the professions universally corrupted, Kozinski argues that we must prepare ourselves spiritually for the Great Tribulation and the arrival of Antichrist. This is a bold book that is unafraid to call out the evil in our world for what it is, and to consider what kind of education is required in the Age of Unreality."

— Dr. David A. Hughes,
author of *"Covid-19," Psychological Operations, and the War for Technocracy, Volume 1* and *Wall Street, the Nazis, and the Crimes of the Deep State*

"Thaddeus Kozinski is a teacher who turns your thinking upside down, destroys the order of your thoughts and insists that there is a better way of putting them together. What he deals with here is the question of evil, which he tells us is not a problem but a mystery. His laboratory sample is the plandemic of 2020. He takes apart this mystery, which so many us have pondered for five years, and shows us that our understandings have been tentative, partial. We need to go deeper into things, he plausibly insists, to go to the centre of all meanings, for that is where the truth about this, and everything, resides. He diagnoses the roots of what has happened in that perversion of freedom, liberalism, an ideology of counterfeit liberty. But he cuts deeper than sociological or ideological analysis, to expose why even Christ's own Church became implicated in the evil-doing. These events, he outlines, are the culmination of Biblical prophecies and warnings, and are therefore to be seen as the inevitable outcome of man's rejection of God. What is happening to the world now is, accordingly, being permitted by God as a means of restoring His authority over his creation. When, in the past five years, we have heard people speak of what has been happening as a 'spiritual war', it has not always been clear what this means. In this book we find the answer: it is ultimately a war declared by men against God, and which is therefore, ultimately, a war declared by man upon himself. This is a book for both the faithful and the faithless, for it speaks to the part of each of us that is eternal, even if in spite of ourselves. When Thaddeus Kozinski proposes as the beginnings of a solution what he calls "existential Christianity," he is acknowledging the linguistic trap into which man has painted himself: he is not God but has abolished God, and so must replace him, even in his total inadequacy. Only in seeing this, can we perceive the error of the totalitarians, and grasp the formula by which to pursue their banishment."

— John Waters,
Thinker, Talker, and Writer

"The world has nowhere come to full consciousness of what happened to us from 2020-2023 under the pretense of mastering the microbial kingdom. They targeted all human life in what amounts to a coup against civilization and its foundational moral and spiritual principles. This is where Thaddeus Kozinski comes in to offer an even deeper analysis that speaks to theological concerns, the replacement of an organic liturgy of life with a manufactured one straight out of the worst dystopian novel. It's no wonder people are in denial. This book reveals the fullness of what happened as a path toward spiritual healing."

— Jeffrey Tucker,
Brownstone Institute

"With clarity, urgency, and profound charity, Thaddeus Kozinski argues that liberalism is the ideological medium of totalitarianism, and correspondingly, that modernity is the historical vessel of the worldly west's collective "perfect possession," that starkest spiritual condition, marked by a hermetic severance (psychic as well as intellectual) from the Divine. From this unfolds the inevitability of an eschatological moment—*our* moment—looming with the horrors of *anomos*, the man of lawlessness: Antichrist, against whom there is no secular or political hope whatsoever. To the scapegoating bloodlust which *anomos* recently unleashed in the modern liberal leviathan, Kozinski responds with a vision of that mercy inhabiting (as he ventures to call it) "the Divine Revelation of evil." In light of which anyone still capable of listening is summoned to observe the only Perfect Sacrifice, and this in humble submission to His cosmic authority and faultless love for us. Which alone reveal the profane blood rites of our satanic elite for what they are, and what they portend: the dread yawning of hell's gates, amid which salvation beckons this last time."

—Thomas Breidenbach,
poet, parapolitical researcher, and
author of *IX XI and the Mysteries of State* (in manuscript)

COVID 19

AND THE

WAR AGAINST REALITY

Thaddeus J. Kozinski, Ph.D.

Foreword by Thomas Breidenbach

En Route Books and Media, LLC
Saint Louis, MO

⊕ENROUTE
Make the time

En Route Books and Media, LLC

5705 Rhodes Avenue

Saint Louis, MO 63109

Contact us at

contactus@enroutebooksandmedia.com

ISBN-13: 979-8-88870-333-5

Library of Congress Control Number: 2025934410

Table of Contents

Foreword

Giorgio Agamben reminds us of the ancient Greek distinction between two forms of life, *zoē* and *bios*, with the latter referring to the manner or way of living, the quality of life and what is proper to it, and the former denoting the biological fact of life itself, or what Agamben calls *bare life*. This he characterizes as that zone of indistinction between man and beast, in which (in Thomas Hobbes' phrase) man is a wolf to man, and wherein Hobbes' state of nature, his war of all against all, stands revealed not only as origin but, too, as destiny.[1] It is, in other words, that decisive characteristic of our sociological present, wherein it resides in varying degrees of potentiality—the more acutely in the modern age, which in its secularization increasingly regards bare life as the only life.

As the Covid-19 era illustrated—with such deadly, obscene, and absurd incessance—bare life's latency within our globalized culture has suddenly worn terrifyingly thin, such that behind the fraying veil of *bios* at least two of the apocalypse's dread horsemen—plague and war—can be seen galloping upon the encroaching horizon of *zoē*. This terror confronts those still attuned to *logos* (in short, meaningful thought) with the dire immanence of a metanarrative hubristically denied by the (post)modern mind: the mythic sacred, and the human sacrificial imperative with which it confronts each and all of us.

---

[1] Agamben, Giorgio. *Homo Sacer: Sovereign Power and Bare Life*. Translated by Daniel Heller-Roazen. (Redwood City, CA: Stanford University Press, 1998), 106.

Faced ineluctably with what Ananda K. Coomaraswamy characterizes as the truth of myth—which as Sallust knew may transcend
its simplistic or literal truth—we find in our sacred narratives and
Tradition, and only in them, the truth our modern world denies, and
which by way of that denial it but verifies. We find, that is, what
Michel Serres understood, that only myth understands history—our
history very much included.

In articulating his theory of "political theology," Carl Schmitt
observes that

> All significant concepts of the modern theory of the state are
> secularized theological concepts not only because of their
> historical development—in which they were transferred
> from theology to the theory of the state, whereby, for exam-
> ple, the omnipotent God became the omnipotent lawgiver—
> but also because of their systematic structure, the recogni-
> tion of which is necessary for a sociological consideration of
> these concepts. The exception in jurisprudence is analogous
> to the miracle in theology. Only by being aware of this anal-
> ogy can we appreciate the manner in which the philosophical
> ideas of the state developed in the last centuries. (Schmitt 36)

What Schmitt terms "the exception" appears as that extralegal
circumstance through which state sovereignty is expressed and
maintained, and by way of which conditions beyond the perceived
effect or purview of the law are dealt with by the sovereign, with
these conditions being determined by the sovereign alone.

However paradoxical, Schmitt's idea of, in essence, *that violation of the law upon which the law is (ultimately) based* is critical in conceptualizing the *parapolitical*, the emerging academic discipline focusing upon the role of elite violence or criminality in the conduct of statecraft. Yet while essential to any theory of the state capable of contextualizing the apparent range of the state's functions—especially those mysterious extralegal or criminal functions which the modern demos are relentlessly propagandized to deny, at the cost of any among them who fail to do so being remorselessly stigmatized—there is something missing in Schmitt's formulation.

And that is what Thaddeus Kozinski's writing redresses. That is, whereas Schmitt articulates a theory of political theology, Kozinski presents a necessary reversal of Schmitt's formulation, offering a *theological politics* drawn from what Kozinski calls "the Catholic actuality," which he, borrowing from the work of D.C. Schindler, defines as "the tradition that synthesized, once and for all, the Greek, the Roman, the Hebrew, the Germanic—all the tributaries of the axial age that came together with Christ." If it was only by peering from politics back toward theology that Schmitt was able dramatically to clarify political philosophy, then it is only by peering at politics from its origin in theology that the nature of the political—and of modern politics in particular—may be fully illuminated.

However belatedly, consider what that illumination reveals about our present political condition. Marked as it is by the concomitant and mutually aggravating factors of: a radical secularization and deregulation of desire; an inherently thermonuclear warmongering now largely emanating from those insisting that desire's deregulation is a form of liberation; a seething internecine hatred between the two prominent political factions of our national family (globalism versus nationalism); and the various forms of psychopathy metastasizing not only at the demotic level (as the tensions just mentioned attest) but also at the level of our political elite as well, as evidenced by the "exceptional" (in the Schmittian sense) measures to which they would appear to have resorted in the face of the mounting crises characterizing the anomic catastrophe in which our western disenchantment is culminating.

All of which marks our parlous return to what the philosopher René Girard (a formative influence on Kozinski) understood as the primitive sacred. Which is to say that we are returned to a consciousness of the mythic realm's reality, having as a culture exchanged the protection afforded alone by Christ's Blood for a counterfeit protection offered within our pagan recrudescence, typified as it is by contemporary versions of antiquity's state-sanctioned desire cults and the mass human sacrificial spectacles that alone inspire the terror and awe through which these cults might cohere, however tenuously or provisionally.

What we find ourselves realizing, in still other words, is that esoteric truth referred to by Socrates in Plato's *Gorgias*:

> You see, I wouldn't wonder that Euripides is saying the truth in
>   these [verses], when he says:
> Who knows whether to live is to die,
> And to die is to live?
> and *we* in reality are perhaps dead. (492e)

We find ourselves, that is, in the underworld, enduring a living death wherein the dire truths of our condition face us with what feels like ruthless blatancy, where (for example) the illicit affair between Aphrodite and Ares—the gods, respectively, of licentiousness and of war—is luridly manifest in the historical reality of our day.

Relatedly, consider the apocalyptic dialectic which the Book of Revelation portrays between the beast and the whore, how the unfoldment of apocalypse entails, in a profane parody of the Divine Family, the sadistic interaction between these two negative masculine and feminine archetypes. These appear in Revelation as what Girard calls mimetic *twins* or *violent doubles*, in that the degradations of the whore appear to incite the hateful and violent turning of the beast against her, even though she had previously ridden the beast. It is difficult not to see in this a portent of the dehumanizing sexual license of our moment lending to a fatal corrosion of sensibility that promises to culminate—upon a sufficient sense of collective crisis, such as an economic collapse and/or the outbreak of global war—in the sort of scapegoating violence that, as Girard so brilliantly warns, human groups default to in what they experience as a sacred search for an order preserving them against collective dissolution and death.

Relevant here is Plato's harrowing vision in the *Republic* of the democratic regime, which culminates in the equality of animals and men—with this appearing (among other associations) as a premonition of certain sexual fetishes attaining prevalence today. According to Plato, despite its love of freedom—or more correctly, as a result of it—democracy engenders tyranny, which appears as a desperate search for that order which democracy had abandoned in its love of freedom. To conflate Western tradition's elucidatory schemas, democracy engenders the whore, who triumphally enters astride the beast of tyranny before that beast hatefully turns and burns the whore with fire. The whore in effect licenses or "mothers" the beast, in that it could not have been born without her, while the beast, in apparent subservience to her initially, at first bears the whore whom it is its destiny to burn.

Given our culture's manifestation of increasingly unregulated desire and the violence that (as our mythic inheritance amply affirms) inevitably attends it, we can only recall, with a certain shudder, what the Romans understood, that Cupid (Greek Eros), while the most beautiful of the gods, is nonetheless the god born for the destruction of the world. Nor can we ignore what tradition instructs is portended by late imperialism's ultimate cult—the cult of victimization, which has claimed the minds of so many in the west. This is especially pertinent given Girard's warning that the last disguise of Satan will be that of the victim, or René Guénon's similar caution that a mark of the end times will be the return of Abel—the vengeful return of the victim. In short, the primordial conflict from which civilization emerges—that between Cain and Abel—engenders that conflict in which it will end, that between Gog and Magog, whose armies now amass in the Armageddon of our own political circumstance.

As we are helped to see by the corrective of theological politics that Kozinski (among others he mentions) articulates, such apparent sovereign exceptions as IX XI and Covid-19 stand revealed not merely as secular equivalents of miracles, but as (in a phrase) "satanic miracles" in which the lives of others are willingly exchanged for a sense of security, with this exchange occurring, in effect, collectively, given the virulence with which so many in modern culture cleave to the lies necessary to these lethal "miracles'" efficacy. What theological politics ultimately exposes, then, is not only the sorcerous nature of the modern state, but the capitulation to state sorcery on the part of the secularized contemporary demos, who appear in Kozinski's analysis as the very thing we are least prepared to acknowledge about ourselves: the perfect subjects of an unprecedented tyranny—or rather, that tyranny finding precedent only within the concluding book of scripture.

With extraordinary candor, urgency, and charity, Kozinski argues that liberalism is the ideological medium of totalitarianism, and correspondingly, that modernity is the historical vessel of the worldly west's collective "perfect possession," that starkest spiritual condition, marked by a hermetic severance, psychic as well as intellectual, from the Divine. From this unfolds the inevitability of an eschatological moment—*our* moment—looming with the horrors of *anomos*, the man of lawlessness: Antichrist, against whom there is no secular or political hope whatsoever.

To the scapegoating bloodlust which *anomos* recently unleashed in the modern liberal leviathan, Kozinski responds with a vision of that mercy inhabiting "the Divine Revelation of evil" (as he ventures to call it), and the compassion to which that vision calls us even, or *especially*, in this late hour. And in light of which anyone still capable of heeding it is summoned to observe the only Perfect Sacrifice, and this in humble submission to His cosmic authority and faultless love for us.

Against the sacrifices of others increasingly defining our frenzied hour, Kozinski clarifies our sacred calling to attest to that hour's forbidden truths, and this at the perpetual risk of the self-sacrifice modeled for us by Socrates, and more ultimately by Christ, Whose Sacrifice alone most fully reveals the profane blood rites of our satanic elite for what they are: the entrance to hell, from which salvation beckons this last time.

—Thomas Breidenbach,
poet, parapolitical researcher,
and author of *IX XI and the Mysteries of State* (in manuscript)

Chapter I

The Warning

Antichrist Rising

The sacred is that which ineluctably holds us in its grip, a reality it is forbidden to eschew or doubt. The sacred is inevitable and inexorable, for it is the divine ground of reality, and to treat it as a mere option, as modernity teaches us to do, is deadly to both the soul and the community of souls. The contemporary worship of "options"—from what brand of high-fructose poison to consume to what gender to adopt—is nothing but defiance of the sacred order of *Logos* antecedent to and authoritative over any of our subjective preferences: "Am I really a creature of this God standing before me, or is He perhaps a creature like me? After all, I did not witness my own creation!" And with that proto-modern gesture of defiance, the Miltonian Lucifer inaugurated his endless rejection of Reality. But what is sometimes *taken* to be sacred, of course, might not actually be so, for counterfeits abound, and we must defy idols at all costs. Indeed, any sacred in opposition to the One, True, Sacred of Jesus Christ and His Church is a lying counterfeit deserving to be smashed to smithereens.

Contemporary society is replete with idols, for it is not in conformity with the Gospel. Indeed, its leaders and reigning ideologies celebrate the four sins that cry to heaven for vengeance: over a bil-

lion legally authorized murdered babies since abortion was first le-
galized in Soviet Russia; the ubiquitous public endorsement of ster-
ilized fornication and sodomy; oligarchic theft through usury, taxes,
and wage slavery; and the physical, psychological, and spiritual oppression of the poor though the same, along with mass-media propaganda, formalized and systematic de-education, and ritualistic,
trauma-based, state-sponsored mind-control events. Thus, everyone, and especially Christians, has a moral obligation to doubt the
counterfeit sacreds that are offered to us for acceptance and worship
by the God-hating puppeteers. From September 2001 until March
2020, the regnant counterfeit was IXXI and the genocidal war of terror it unleashed, resulting in millions of murders, a traumatized,
brainwashed, and anemic populous, and an incipient globalist totalitarianism. In 2020 we were given the "Covid-19 pandemic," and
compared to the scope and depth of its horrors, the evil of IXXI pales
in comparison.

Now, lest the reader misunderstand, by "the Covid-19 pandemic" I do not mean any actual disease or pandemic by that name.
For, as every bit of common-sense and scientific evidence, as well as
the in-between-the-lines admissions of today's principalities and
powers (WHO, CDC, NIH, WEF, etc.), make abundantly clear,
there was no Covid-19 pandemic.[1] Instead, it was the installation,
under the cloud of a medical hoax, of a new global and totalitarian
religion commanding and coercing our obedience to its Great Lie,
to fear and hatred of all that is true, good, and beautiful.[2] Its liturgy

---

[1] See the work of Denis Rancourt, https://denisrancourt.sub-stack.com/p/
what-the-declared-pandemic-was-and.

[2] The most comprehensive and accurate book on the real nature of the event

included psychotically fearful, masked zombies celebrating their forced isolation and torture[3], the destruction of their livelihood, the shutdown of the food supply chain, and a "New Normal" resembling nothing so much as The Hunger Games.

But is not the sacred an extinct relic of our benighted, superstitious, medieval past? In truth, the hell-on-earth that emerged in 2020 is precisely what any society must have when the true sacred is replaced with a false one, even if under the cover of a godless and nihilistic denial of the objective existence of any sacred at all—well, other than "my choice."[4] Reality Himself, Whom we should fear with holy reverence, the omnipotent, omnipresent, and invisible True and Only Sacred, namely, The Eternal Father, His Son the Lord Jesus Christ, and the Holy Spirit Who is their Eternal Love, has been rejected and replaced by Unreality, a fake omnipotent, omnipresent, and invisible "virus" (literally, an existing *nothing* with no substance of its own) that we were commanded to fear with unholy terror or suffer perpetual mockery, ostracization, and even death.[5] And then

---

is David A. Hughes, *"Covid-19," Psychological Operations, and the War for Technocracy, Volume 1,* (Cham, Switzerland, Palgrave Macmillan, 2024), Available for download at https://link. springer.com/book/10.1007/978-3-031-41850-1#bibliographic-information.

[3] See the work of podcaster and journalist, "Amazing Polly," who made it clear in 2020 that the Covid "regulations" fit perfectly the Amnesty International definition of torture and Biderman's "Chart of Coercion": https://www.bitchute.com/video/3yk3xezML8Q/.

[4] https://www.youtube.com/watch?v=HeTjZcylb_8.

[5] https://www.sydneycriminallawyers.com.au/blog/man-has-seizure-after-being-arrested-for-not-wearing-a-mask/

we were all anointed, else be cast into the outer darkness, with a sacramental "vaccine" that was nothing other than a disease-delivery system inserted right into our DNA.[6]

How can we account for this hell-on-earth, overseen by psychopathic technocrats and their willing slaves, and orchestrated by demons and their occultist worshipers on earth? This was something unimaginable before 2020. I have been racking my brain for years trying to answer this question, and this is the best I can come up with. God is mercifully revealing to the world the naked and brutal reality of our collective choice, both personally and corporately, to live in opposition to Him, to choose unreality, knowingly and deliberately. This unreality is administered to the world by globalist elites using the latest propaganda technology and a panopticon-like surveillance and censorship apparatus. The effectiveness of their creation of unreality can be gauged by the success of their two-fold Big Lie, namely, that there was a deadly pandemic, and that asymptomatic transmission could ever be a real thing, a lie that gave these psychopaths total control of the world economy as well as all the major institutions of governance and culture.

Due especially to those in positions of responsibility and leadership embracing this lie, or at least not opposing it, but also to the masses who have irresponsibly deferred to these, we found and still find ourselves in a seemingly inescapable matrix of inverted reality, with meaninglessness masking itself as conviction, fear as love, isolation as solidarity, destitution as generosity, poison as medicine, ideology as science, propaganda as fact, abuse as justice. But why

---

[6]https://rumble.com/v521lph-dr.-sherri-tenpenny-the-mrna-vaccines-are-literally-death-by-our-own-govern.html.

have so many accepted a lie over the truth? I don't think the answer is just the ubiquity and sophistication of the propaganda. Common sense and personal experience make it patently obvious that there was no pandemic (other than the deliberate harm and death that was caused by the public authorities), just a psychological torture operation, not to mention that the Elites have admitted it quite plainly (you just have to listen to what they are saying in between the lies—they have admitted that the Covid-19 fatality rate, for example, was comparable to a bad seasonal flu, and this even with so many deaths from other causes falsely attributed to Covid). There was and is a widespread and mysterious yearning for these self-destructive lies.

Insofar as the West embraced Liberalism, i.e., the privatization of Truth and Goodness—practical atheism—we have already been living in unreality for centuries. The hard physical and legal totalitarianism we are now experiencing is but the flip side of the soft psychological and spiritual totalitarianism that has made us ready and willing to accept and even embrace the former. The empty shrine of the American idol of "the freedom of religion" was never actually empty, though the diabolical entities inhabiting it and manipulating our souls were then well disguised. Now, not so much. The same siren voices of authority pre-Covid that were instructing the left-minded to "question authority" and "keep religion out of the bedroom," and the right-souled to "kill the terrorists over there before they kill us over here," and "support our troops" commanded us in 2020 slowly to suffocate ourselves and allow our livelihoods, communities, and families to be destroyed—and we listened and obeyed like the good Americans we are. After all, we're free! We don't have an "established religion" like those ragheads over there and those papists way back when. We're enlightened! And that's why we lined up to be injected with a poisonous DNA-changing technology at the behest of senile pedophiles like Joe Biden, frauds like Anthony Fauci, and genocidal maniacs like Bill Gates. Individual liberty, the rule of law, and the separation of Church and state quickly became individual self-enslavement, the rule of psychopathic will, and Church-approved state apotheosis (the American Bishops as a whole seemed almost gleeful to give over their shepherd staffs to moronic and brutal bureaucrats—wear your mask!). It was never freedom and autonomy and self-government, was it? It was always obedience to the Sacred State and the demonic voice speaking through it. When that voice was seductive and libertine and mammon-friendly, then it seemed like freedom and bliss to obey it, but in 2020 it showed its true face, the face of pure hatred, control, and murder, and we must still obey, even though we know that it is leading us to hell.

As I say, I have been racking my brain trying to figure out how we can get out of this seemingly inexorable spiral to complete enslavement and unimaginable horror. My conclusion is that we cannot do it ourselves. We are in a collective state of perfect possession. There are saints among us, of course, who have remained immune to the leprous spiritual disease, and these are suffering tremendously and heroically for us as victim souls; and there are many who are doing their best to resist the evil and insanity, though I am afraid many are doing it in the name of the very demons they think to be fighting—"bodily autonomy," "individual liberty," "religious freedom," etc. The only solution is for the whole world to be given a clear vision of reality, for Satan to be blinded if only for a moment, and for everyone everywhere to see themselves as God sees them.

Such an event is coming, very soon if the consensus of Catholic mystics and visionaries are right, and it is called the Miracle of the Illumination of all Consciences or The Warning. Perhaps the only thing we can do right now is to prepare our souls for it. This should be our priority.

What Plato Could Have Taught Us in 2020

Plato taught us that the purpose of life is to know, love, and serve the Good, which is at once Reality itself, its source, and the power by which we know and love it. Plato also taught us that, as humans are communal, they know, love, and serve the Good together in communities, especially the larger community of the polis or city. For Plato and the *philosophia perennis*, Reality is the Good and the Good is Reality, and as such the foundation and purpose of both personal and political life.

But what is Reality, and how do we know it? No one grappled with this question more deeply than Plato, giving us the classic distinction between what appears and what is. The Good is both What Is and the perfect self-awareness of What Is, and so the distinction doesn't apply to It. But you and I are not the Good, and this otherness puts us at some distance from it, in the space between which, as it were, the Good makes its appearance. The whole point of Platonism is to reduce this distance as much as possible, such that for all intents and purposes, we become one with the Good and thus with Reality. When the philosophers who are to rule the city have obtained this unity through rigorous formation and years of contemplation, they order the city so that those living within it are enabled to become as united with the Real and the Good as possible. Otherwise, as Plato makes clear, tyrants, those who put their desires in the place of the Good and their dictates in the place of Reality, will rule a city of unreality unto self-destruction.

Many people today, particularly the religiously inclined, still agree with Plato that knowing and loving Reality and the Good is the purpose of life, but not many think that political life and social order should be based upon spiritual or even moral reality. Liberalism (in both the classical and late-modern versions) is responsible for this change, as it teaches that the purpose of politics is not to help make people virtuous, know the truth and love the good, and mediate the authority of God, but to provide a secure, morally and religiously neutral "space" by providing the economic and legal (free-market exchange, constitutional law) and communal (family, school, church, etc.) resources by which individuals can freely work out for themselves the difference between appearance and reality and choose to live according to their conclusions without external coercion or even social pressure. People in political power are not authorized to impose their view of the Good and the Real on everyone else, which is what we do not like about the bad, pre-liberal old days. It is not that it would not be a great thing if we all somehow came to an agreement on the highest good and the most real, but that would have to occur through the totally free pursuit of truth by individuals. And even if happened, no established religion or confessional political order could ever be set up again. The secular, pluralistic city is the best one, we know now, for it secures the blessings of liberty and freedom for all requiring only a modicum of shared principles, such as not killing each other over disagreements about the Good and the Real, educational and economic opportunity for all, and not taking other people's stuff. Plato helped us to recognize the connection between the search for the truth about the Good and political peace and happiness, but he went too far when he authorized the political community to establish and impose the Good on itself. No one can be forced to move from appearance to Reality.

But if Reality and the Good is not something we want imposed on us by our rulers, why is it that in March of 2020, we let them do just that? Suddenly, whatever the medical "experts" and "authorities" declared to be reality was reality, at that time, the most deadly global pandemic in human history. And what they declared to be good was good: the shutdown of all social and economic life, social isolation, wearing a mask, and, later, mandated injections. The philosopher-kings also made sure that all people in the world rejected any appearances to the contrary of their declarations, with money, moral accolades, and prestige given to the reality-knowers, and sanctions, demonization, and cancellation for the appearance-lovers. Why did we allow our social and political order to regress to the Middle Ages? Did everyone suddenly re-read Book V of Plato's *Republic*, in which the absurd details of a theocracy of the Good are ironically laid out, and have a conversion experience?

The short answer is fear. It seems that fear can bring out truth, and the truth that emerged in 2020 is that the liberal adventure of "choose your own good" was always nothing but a facade. As long as nothing life-threatening was at stake, the postmodernist play-acting of private bourgeois self-creation and the secularist public agnosticism about Reality and the Good could continue along. IXXI was a significant interruption to the liberal status quo, after which the fear of terrorism saw our ecumenical non-judgmentalism and liberal tolerance morph into a fundamentalist theological crusade against pure evil—with bombs. After the buildings blew up, millions of frightened American children (adults who regressed) were initiated into Reality by their President-Father. Just like today, all dissent from the government-media narrative was forbidden and punished, with agreement rewarded. But in 2001, secular life in America (apart from airports, perhaps) essentially remained the same: the Good/Real was still a private matter. And though on IXXI geopolitical reality was dictated to us from on high, there was still much of the Good and True that we were still permitted to work out for ourselves. As long as "we killed them over there so they wouldn't kill us over here," we were free in our cities, our homes, and in our bodies, and so we were happy with the liberal status quo.

But the 2001 episode of medieval atavism was only a prelude to the full-scale regression of the entire globe in 2020. If fear brings out truth, pathological fear is magisterial. Prefaced by an incessant onslaught of horror propaganda, beginning in March of 2020, we were initiated from on high not only into the new political reality of "the new normal" but also into the new physical reality: Every air molecule in the whole world was now toxic (except the air molecules in the restaurant or plane as soon as you took off your mask to eat and drink). Our healthy, non-symptomatic neighbor's very bodily existence would certainly kill us if we didn't interpose six feet and a piece of cloth. Staying inside one's home and shutting down the in-person economy was the only way to avoid certain death. And every child on earth needed to be injected with an untested experimental drug (even though children were not dying from the disease, the drug did not prevent or cure the disease, and the drug was killing more people than the disease). Did I forget to mention that the human immune system no longer existed in 2020? Yes, we obeyed Reality as it was revealed to us day by day by the medical priests and bureaucratic bishops. We listened and believed because we wanted to know the True Good and the Really Real, and we wanted to know it together. C. J. Hopkins:

> The New Normals — i.e., those still wearing masks outdoors, shrieking over meaningless "cases," bullying everyone to get "vaccinated," and collaborating with the segregation of the "Unvaccinated" — are not behaving the way they're behaving because they are stupid. They are behaving that way because they're living in a new "reality" that has been created for them over the course of several years by a massive official propaganda campaign, the most extensive and effective in the history of propaganda.[7]

It is well known that people in a psychotic state of fear will believe anything, no matter how absurd and destructive, if it promises to give them a way out of the torturing fear. Every would-be totalitarian knows this, and that is why totalitarianism is most effectively ushered in by a mass trauma event followed by an arbitrary assignment of blame, a scapegoating campaign, and a recipe for fear mitigation. If you follow reality by first believing *this* horror story (now

---

[7] C.J. Hopkins, "The Propaganda War (And How to Fight It)," *CJ Hopkins*, 19 July 2021, https://cjhopkins.substack.com/p/the-propaganda-war-and-how-to-fight

you have an object for the free-floating anxiety caused), scapegoating *these* people (now you belong to the community of the righteous), and following *these* mandates (now you have the cure), your loneliness, fear, and guilt will cease. But I think there is a deeper explanation for the transformation of so many postmodern relativists into medieval dogmatists. And here we return to Plato.

Human beings are indeed ordered to the Good and the True, and we are ordered to these by and in community. We crave to know and love and celebrate reality, to live within it and for it, even to give our lives for it, and we want most of all to do these things *together*. We want the Good for ourselves and others, and we want it with others, for, like reality, the Good cannot be enjoyed alone. Reality, after all, is a common good, one that increases and deepens the more people know, love, and share in it. What we want most of all is for our political community to express, authorize, and be founded upon the reality of the good, for we know intuitively that if it is founded on mere human will, however apparently benevolent or democratic, it will tyrannize us. Aristotle expresses the Platonic insight:

> When the community made up of several villages is complete it is then a city, possessing the limit of every self-sufficiency, practically speaking, and though it originates for the sake of life it exists for the sake of the good life. Consequently, every city is by nature, if, that is, the first communities also are. For the city is the end of those communities and nature is an end, since we say that a thing's nature is the sort of thing it is when its generation has been completed (as in the case of a human being, a horse, or a house). Further, that

for the sake of which something is, or its end, is best and self-sufficiency is both an end and best... By nature, then, the drive towards such a community exists in everyone; but the first to set one up is responsible for very great goods. For as human beings are the best of all animals when perfected, so they are the worst when divorced from law and right.[8]

"Right" and "law" are common goods that cannot be adequately established or fully possessed by individuals, families, or even villages. These perfecting goods are only found in the larger and more complex *polis*, and, as Aristotle says, a man who does not live in a polis, or does not need to, is either a beast or a god. But in liberalism, "right" and "law" are not based upon the Good and Reality, for they are mere contractual edicts expressing nothing more than human will. Liberalism's privatization of the Good not only "divorces us from law and right," thus making us the "worst of animals," but also makes us crave reality-based law and good-expressing right.

In the absence of a nationally or globally coordinated psychological operation of terror and torture, citizens of liberal regimes tend to fixate on their free-floating anxiety, assuage their loneliness, and satisfy their inexorable desire for a communally shared reality and an authoritative good by joining together in worship (sometimes authentic religious worship, but also the cults of career, sport, money-making, shopping, etc.). For the saintly among us, who being god-like do not need the polis as much as others, they are perfected well enough by the reality that they know through Divine Revelation and

---

[8] *The Politics of Aristotle,* Translated by Peter Simpson, (Chapel Hill: University of North Carolina Press, 1997), 29-33.

the Tao, that is, without requiring the political publicization of the Good, with their anxiety and loneliness and guilt purged by their intimate relationship with God. But the vast majority of us need a polis as well as a church, one that unites us, not in an isolated and isolating, individualistic pursuit of happiness, but in the communal enjoyment of happiness, in the knowledge, love, and celebration of the Good in the Real.

The Roman Catholic Church is a polis, indeed, the best one, and it is the perfect model for all other polises. But there is nature as well as grace, reason as well as faith, the temporal as well as the spiritual, and we are political animals as much as religious ones, citizens of the City of Man and, by grace, the City of God. In any event, it is not clear that the Church herself (in her human element) has not become a servant of the totalitarian polis. An official Vatican conference was held in May of 2021 that supported the injection of the entire global population with a gene-altering serum. Not to mention their willing closing of their Churches, refusing to hear confessions or give Last Rites, mandating masks and social distancing, and even using parishes as injection sites. Here we have the very custodians and mediators of ultimate reality, the Bishops of the Catholic Church, renouncing their sacred vocation and embracing a counterfeit reality. They must have been starving for the Good and the True even more than the rest of us.

The totalitarianism to which we were subjected in 2020 is best explained as the "return of the repressed," and as we know from horror movies, the form this return takes is always a monster. Observing the totalitarian monster birthed from the ontological and spiritual vacuum of liberalism rampaging around the globe claiming to be reality incarnate, and the billions following the monster blindly as he approached the cliff, we can see just how powerful our need is for institutions and authorities to be based upon reality and the good. When Christ is dethroned, Antichrist is waiting in the wings, and we would rather have him than nothing. Literal global insanity was unleashed due to this primordial spiritual need having been repressed for so long and so extensively, giving birth to existential fear now grown to pathological levels, satiated and exacerbated by a counterfeit reality promulgated by a counterfeit authority offering a counterfeit savior from a counterfeit evil.

In short, the last four years are perhaps *the* demonstrative proof that Plato was right, though he did not know that the Good would eventually come down from heaven and live in a backwater town somewhere east of Athens. And since we know that the Good and the Real is Jesus Christ, perhaps in 2020 we were given demonstrative proof of Catholicism as well. Pope Pius XI:

> With God and Jesus Christ, we said, excluded from political life, with authority derived not from God but from man, the very basis of that authority has been taken away, because the chief reason of the distinction between ruler and subject has been eliminated. The result is that human society is tottering to its fall, because it has no longer a secure and solid foundation.[9]

---

[9] Pope Pius XI, *Quas Primas*, The Holy See, 11 Dec. 1925, n. 18, https://www.vatican.va/content/pius-xi/en/encyclicals/documents/hf_p-xi_enc_11121925_quas-primas.html.

From Liberal Democracy to Global Totalitarianism

> An excessive desire for liberty at the expense of every-
> thing else is what undermines democracy and leads to the
> demand for tyranny.
>
> —Plato[10]

In a 2021 lecture at Notre Dame[11], Alasdair MacIntyre argued
that the claims and conceptions of universal and inalienable human
dignity as reflected in documents such as the 1948 United Nations'
Universal Declaration of Human Rights and in various post-war European constitutions are puzzling, since this dignity requires a duty
of respect to everyone just for being human, no matter their behavior or character, so Stalin the mass murderer has as much dignity
and deserves as much respect as Mother Teresa. Aquinas' view
of *dignitas* as interpreted by Charles De Koninick[12] is a challenge to
this view, for it assigns human dignity, not to the mere fact of being
human, but to end to which we are called, which is supernatural,
union with God, which might not be attained due to one's choices
on earth against those common goods which enable our attainment
of the supernatural end, and so human *dignitas* could be lost. According to this view, which is founded on the end to which humans
are called and the virtue of justice, not the mere fact of being human
and an ambiguous and philosophically ungrounded human dignity,

---

[10] Plato, *The Republic*, trans. Desmond Lee (London: Penguin, 2007), 562c.

[11] Alasdair MacIntyre, "Human Dignity: A Puzzling and Possibly Dangerous
Idea?" (lecture, University of Notre Dame, de Nicola Center for Ethics and Culture, YouTube, https://www.youtube.com/watch?v=5s8pJ5vRmXg).

the 20th-century concept of human dignity is much too individualistic, and because it is not based in justice and the common good, only can provide negative prescriptions against the undignified treatment of humans. It is unable to provide positive prescriptions that enable persons to obtain the common goods and the virtues they need to attain their supernatural end. For MacIntyre, we need to speak of human dignity in terms of justice, what we owe to each other for the sake of enabling persons to attain their personal and common goods and final end, which is the knowledge and love of God in this life and the next.

I would like to use MacIntyre's lecture as a springboard to talk about the current situation of the world. Since March of 2020, we have suffered an all-out, deliberate, and planned assault on both human dignity and justice. To see this, I cite the *Catechism of the Catholic Church*'s section on "Respect for the Dignity of Human Persons"[13] which is a kind of synthesis of the Thomistic justice and common good-oriented and the modern rights and dignity-oriented views, presenting a set of both negative proscriptions and positive prescriptions for what this respect requires. It will be shown that every one of these has been violated to the core under the pretext of public health and a "viral pandemic." I think the reason for the success of this assault, waged by billionaire globalist elites and the Department of Defense,[14] with the complicity and cooperation of national governments, was the lack of popular resistance to it, indeed,

---

[13] *Catechism of the Catholic Church*, 2nd ed. (Vatican City: Libreria Editrice Vaticana, 1997), §§1928–1942.

[14] See the work of Katherine Watt: https://bailiwicknews.substack.com/?utm_source=substack&utm_medium=web&utm_campaign=substack_profile.

the popular acceptance and even celebration of it. And I think the reason for this malignant effect upon souls is the ideology of secular liberalism.

David Walsh in *Politics of the Person as the Politics of Being*[15] argues that the secular liberalism that produced the 1948 United Nations' *Universal Declaration of Human Rights* and various post-war European constitutions, although not founded on any particular theology or metaphysics or anthropology, indeed, not founded on anything other than a consensus and commitment to the rights and dignity of the human person, is worth preserving and celebrating for its wonderful achievements. He writes:

> Liberal constitutions have emerged from the competition of modern political forms to outlast and surpass all rivals. Not only did they supersede monarchical and aristocratic forms to establish commercial republics, but they have overcome the far more formidable challenges posed by collectivist and authoritarian rivals in the last and present centuries. Despite their weakness and unpreparedness, liberal democracies found within themselves the resources necessary to defeat fascism and persevere through the long confrontation with communism. Now they stand as the exemplars not only of economic and political success but as the model of moral legitimacy the world over, even as they are challenged by the lingering assertion of authoritarian models. No higher aspiration prevails in the contemporary world than to create a

---

[15] David Walsh, *Politics of the Person as the Politics of Being* (Notre Dame, IN: University of Notre Dame Press, 2015).

political order that is derived from and ordered toward the preservation of individual dignity and respect. The moral and political authority of liberal democratic forms may be ironic, given their own inner self-doubt, but it can hardly be denied as a global reality.[16]

Well, the irony, I am afraid, is much deeper than mere "inner self-doubt." In the section on the Fifth Commandment, under the heading of "Respect for the Dignity of Persons," the *Catechism of the Catholic Church* presents five norms that must be obeyed and upheld by persons and societies. Far from fulfilling these norms, virtually all the governments of liberal democracies in the world, those with "no higher aspiration . . . than to create a political order that is derived from and ordered to the preservation of individual dignity and respect," have attacked the dignity of persons on a scale never before seen in human history. The *Catechism* states:

Respect for the souls of others: scandal:

> Therefore, they are guilty of scandal who establish laws or social structures leading to the decline of morals and the corruption of religious practice, or to "social conditions that, intentionally or not, make Christian conduct and obedience to the Commandments difficult and practically impossible." This is also true of business leaders who make

---

[16] Walsh, *Politics of the Person as the Politics of Being*, 224-225.

rules encouraging fraud, teachers who provoke their children to anger, or manipulators of public opinion who turn it away from moral values.

Respect for health:

Concern for the health of its citizens requires that society help in the attainment of living-conditions that allow them to grow and reach maturity: food and clothing, housing, health care, basic education, employment, and social assistance.

If morality requires respect for the life of the body, it does not make it an absolute value. It rejects a neo-pagan notion that tends to promote the cult of the body, to sacrifice everything for its sake, to idolize physical perfection and success at sports.

Respect for the person and scientific research:

Research or experimentation on the human being cannot legitimate acts that are in themselves contrary to the dignity of persons and to the moral law. The subjects' potential consent does not justify such acts. Experimentation on human beings is not morally legitimate if it exposes the subject's life or physical and psychological integrity to disproportionate or avoidable risks. Experimentation on human beings does not conform to the dignity of the person

if it takes place without the informed consent of the subject
or those who legitimately speak for him.

Respect for bodily integrity:

Kidnapping and hostage taking bring on a reign of terror; by means of threats they subject their victims to intolerable pressures. They are morally wrong. Terrorism threatens, wounds, and kills indiscriminately; it is
gravely against justice and charity. Torture which uses
physical or moral violence to extract confessions, punish
the guilty, frighten opponents, or satisfy hatred is contrary
to respect for the person and for human dignity. Except
when performed for strictly therapeutic medical reasons,
directly intended amputations, mutilations, and steriliza-
tions performed on innocent persons are against the moral
law.

Respect for the dead:

The dying should be given attention and care to help
them live their last moments in dignity and peace. They will
be helped by the prayer of their relatives, who must see to
it that the sick receive at the proper time the sacraments
that prepare them to meet the living God.

How have the "models of moral legitimacy" called liberal democracies lived up to these five norms? In March of 2020, we witnessed the emergence of a global totalitarianism the scope and gravity of which has no precedent in history, replete with monstrous scandals (laws allowing abortion mills and liquor stores to stay open while schools and churches are shut down), domestic terrorism (fear-porn propaganda and state-sanctioned violence against peaceful protesters), horrific medical experimentation with no informed consent, and a wanton disrespect for health (outlawing effective life-saving medicine, mandating immune-system destroying injections), bodily integrity (useless and harmful masks and vaccinations known to cause sterilization and death), and the dead (forcing the dying to die alone in nursing homes and hospitals).

Reiner Fuellmich[17] has made a powerful case that what should be called the *plandemic* was the greatest crime against humanity ever committed, essentially a global medical experiment and military operation ordered to genocidal depopulation and sterilization, Big Pharma profits, and totalitarian, economic and political control. We must add to this the psychological devastation, with billions transformed overnight into brainwashed, abused, degraded, and dehumanized persons through what has been diagnosed by competent psychologists as mass-formation psychosis.[18] What we witnessed in the very liberal democracies that according to Walsh are "the exemplars not only of economic and political success but as the model of moral legitimacy the world over" was a global mass terror campaign

---

[17] "Home," *Grand Jury*, accessed December 14, 2024, https://grand-jury.net/.
[18] Mattias Desmet, *The Psychology of Totalitarianism* (New York: Chelsea Green Publishing, 2022).

of fear and torture in which millions consented to, or at least did not widely and forcefully resist, a global economic shutdown leading to millions of deaths, the devastation of national economies, and the destruction of the property-owning middle class. This shutdown included deprivation of fundamental human rights, including the setting up of literal concentration camps for the unvaccinated, the physically and psychologically damaging and medically useless masking of whole populations, including young children, and the insane program of injecting every living human being with an untested, gene-altering serum, what we now know was a bioweapon and designed as such,[19] all for a disease that according to the actual numbers was and is for the vast majority of people no more fatal than the flu.

In America in particular, we have also seen the cultural decadence and scandal of television shows glorifying the sexualization of pre-teens and death games for sport, and the wholescale rejection of the natural law with the ever-increasing celebration and normalization of abortion, sodomy, and transgenderism. Marxist critical-race theory has fueled the scapegoating of non-minority populations as intrinsically racist, with full permission given for mass rioting and looting, and the FBI has declared parents to be domestic terrorists just for raising questions about the curriculum and policies at their children's schools at school board meetings. And let's not forget the US support for the out-in-the-open Israeli genocide of Palestinians,

---

[19] Bailiwick News, "Orientation for New Readers," *Bailiwick News (Substack)*, accessed December 14, 2024, https://bailiwicknews.substack.com/p/orientation-for-new-readers.

according to its own sacrificial logic and nationalist idolatry. Marvin and Ingle:

> To concede that nationalism is a religion is to expose it to challenge, to make it just the same as sectarian religion. By explicitly denying that our national symbols and duties are sacred, we shield them from competition with sectarian symbols. In so doing, we embrace the ancient command not to speak the sacred, ineffable name of god. The god is inexpressible, unsayable, unknowable, beyond language. But that god may not be refused when it calls for sacrifice.[20]

Again: "The first principle of every religious system is that only the deity may kill. The state, which does kill, allows whoever accepts these terms to exist, to pursue their own beliefs and call themselves what they like in the process.[21] As Cavanaugh puts it: "In other words, a basic principle of American openness is that you may confess on your lips any god you like, provided you are willing to kill for America."[22]

David Walsh writes: "Whatever benefits might accrue to the whole society, they are not worth gaining if it means the sacrifice of

---

[20] Carolyn Marvin and David W. Ingle, *Blood Sacrifice and the Nation: Totem Rituals and the American Flag* (Cambridge: Cambridge University Press, 1999), 770.

[21] Ibid., 19.

[22] William T. Cavanaugh, "The Empire of the Empty Shrine: American Imperialism and the Church," *Journal for the Theology of Culture*, Summer 2006, 15.

its humblest member. We simply know that we do not wish to belong to any society that would live at the expense of its most vulnerable members."[23] If this is true, why did the majority of citizens around the world acquiesce so quickly and easily to measures that sacrificed their most vulnerable members? The economic victims of the lockdowns and school shutdowns were primarily the lower classes and children, and masking children for hours on end is literal torture. The Injections have killed more children than they saved, they are known to be made from aborted fetuses—and children are virtually immune from any harm from the virus. Can this be seen as anything but living at the expense of the most vulnerable? The autism rate is now 1 in 36 children. This is completely insane, and undoubtedly due to the increase in mandatory childhood vaccines—72 now! We are sacrificing our children to the new Moloch of "public health."

However one explains the present totalitarianism (and if you deny that we are now living under globalist totalitarianism, you are beyond the reach of argument), it cannot be denied that it emerged from the cultural and political soil of what we call liberal democracies. There are only two explanations for this. One is that a revolution happened, one in complete opposition to those secular, enlightened, liberal principles and practices that are truly ordered by and to the dignity of and respect for the human person. Marxists or fascists or psychos have infiltrated the liberal sanctuary and profaned it. The other explanation is that the totalitarianism we are now undergoing is logically entailed by the very principles and practices of liberal democracy, which are not ordered by and to the dignity of

---

[23] Walsh, *Politics of the Person as the Politics of Being*, 16.

and respect for the human person, but only claim to be. I think the latter explanation is the more plausible one.

Chad Pecknold:

> The progressive civic-religious regime is very dangerous sort
> of pseudo-integralism, which is to say an inverted parody of
> Christianity. The good news is that this has exposed some-
> thing. It has exposed the lie that a religiously neutral polity
> is possible at all. For all of human history, political and social
> order has sought religious unity precisely because religion is
> a precept of the natural law — we cannot do without it. The
> liberal dream of religious neutrality is an anomaly of a couple
> hundred years that is simply not natural, and so it's simply
> not sustainable.[24]

The empty shrine of liberalism was never really empty, as all political orders seek religious unity, even if the religion is a satanic one
in opposition to all that is true, good, and beautiful. We have enshrined arbitrary power and meaningless, directionless, anarchic
freedom, and we are all supposed to have this power and freedom,
but who are "we"? From the perspective of the liberal state in which
the Good is privatized and Truth is perspectival, man is an intrinsically meaningless, directionless, anarchic vector of force (hopefully
not getting in the way of other men), determining his personal
meaning and direction of life by his own will and choices. But that

---

[24] Chad Pecknold, "The Religious Nature of the City," *Postliberal Order*, Jan 24, 2022, https://www.postliberalorder.com/p/the-religious-nature-of-the-city.

all changed in March of 2020. Suddenly we were vectors, not of free choice, but of deadly disease, and we were not permitted to think or act otherwise. Since, according to liberalism there is no God-im-aged-and-ordained teleological human nature and person under-neath the state-imposed vector assignments, or if there is, it cannot be recognized by the State (for the State is proudly a metaphysical, moral, and theological moron); but since the State is in absolute charge of providing, defining, managing, and enforcing personal and group rights, when the State changed the vector denomination from freedom to disease, and forced us all to cover our faces and await mandatory injections under house arrest, there was really nothing we could say or do about it. "If you can't beat 'em, join em" describes the Stockholm syndrome that ensued, with billions of free-dom-loving people all over the world celebrating their enslavement, and scapegoating the minority who resisted it.

DC Schindler:

> Liberalism represents a transformation of human nature from the ground up; it is an extraction of human nature, root and branch, from the actual tradition in which it is embed-ded, so as to enable a truly radical re-interpretation of every dimension of human existence. . . . We propose that there is literally nothing good about liberalism per se—there is noth-ing good about it because, first of all and according to its es-sence, it is as total a rejection of Christianity as is possible, and, moreover, by its nature it is parasitical, something un-

real in itself in the strict metaphysical sense of being priva-tive, insofar as it is founded in a potency that asserts itself over actuality: it is not a reality, as we have seen, but a nega-tion of reality, or perhaps a contrived conspiracy to negate reality. To put this in an extreme formulation, understand-ing evil in the ontological sense of the privation of goodness, we could say that liberalism is evil as a political form.[25]

Insofar as liberalism succeeds in privatizing the good and thereby rendering metaphysical and moral reality purely subjective (and the technocratic manipulation of perceptions has contributed much to this success), its citizens are habituated—imagination, memory, intellect, body, soul, and spirit—accordingly, so that ob-jective reality itself becomes an empty vessel, nothing but the pure potency of "options" to be filled with arbitrary desires and idiosyn-cratic personal preferences, with the strongest ones of the moment (or the most ruthless and cunning group) always winning out. What this amounts to is a "free" populace habituated to be literally out of their minds because cut off from the Logos, the Tao, God. Hannah Arendt was prophetic, and I think her words apply to our day even more than they did to hers.

The ideal subject of totalitarian rule is not the convinced Nazi or the convinced Communist, but people for whom the

---

[25] D.C. Schindler, "What Is Liberalism?" *The Imaginative Conservative*, Au-gust 11, 2023, https://theimaginativeconservative.org/2023/08/what-is-liberal-ism-dc-schindler.html.

distinction between fact and fiction (i.e., the reality of experience) and the distinction between true and false (i.e., the standards of thought) no longer exist.[26]

My thesis is simple: The only plausible explanation for the totalitarianism we have witnessed and which will soon be reactivated with another manufactured crisis is that we citizens of so-called liberal democracies have become the ideal subjects for it. MacIntyre was right. Unless we ground the dignity of the human person in terms of justice, the justice we owe to persons due to their being created in the image and likeness of God and called to communion with Him, we have no rationally compelling reasons for respecting the dignity of persons. But I will go further than MacIntyre to say that unless the political order is explicitly and constitutively ordered to the supernatural end and universal common good of persons, God as revealed by and in Jesus Christ, it cannot adequately provide the common goods of family, workplace, school, and local and ecclesial community, along with the virtues needed for the flourishing of such communities and the securing of such goods. It must thus counterfeit man's supernatural end and universal common good, replacing it with the subhuman, unnatural end of "freedom," but then, logically, (as Plato showed in Book VIII of the *Republic*) enslavement to the most ruthless and powerful in a collectivist and idolatrous worship of state power under totalitarian rule--the annihilation of human dignity. The liberty we all collectively worshipped pre-Covid was already an enslaving, unjust, and self-destructive one,

---

[26] Hannah Arendt, *The Origins of Totalitarianism* (New York: Harcourt, 1951), 474.

but it remained hidden from most. Now it is undeniable and out in the open, though many still cannot see it, and perhaps never will.

It was the Worst of Times

Never has the individual been so completely delivered up to a blind collectivity, and never have men been less capable, not only of subordinating their actions to their thoughts, but even of thinking. Such terms as oppressors and oppressed, the idea of classes—all that sort of thing is near to losing all meaning, so obvious are the impotence and distress of all men in the face of the social machine, which has become a machine for breaking hearts and crushing spirits, a machine for manufacturing irresponsibility, stupidity, corruption, slackness and, above all, dizziness.[27]

It was the best of times, it was the worst of times, it was the age of wisdom, it was the age of foolishness, it was the epoch of belief, it was the epoch of incredulity, it was the season of light, it was the season of darkness, it was the spring of hope, it was the winter of despair.[28]

---

[27] Simone Weil, *The Need for Roots: Prelude to a Declaration of Duties Towards Mankind* (London: Routledge, 1952), 347.

[28] Charles Dickens, *A Tale of Two Cities* (London: Chapman and Hall, 1859), 1.

The best social and political order is the one whereby it is easiest to know truth, adore beauty, and love goodness, especially the highest, most sublime, and best truths, beauties, and goods. This is so because the purpose of life is to attain holiness of soul. Not to mention that truth, beauty, and goodness is the earthly trinity mirroring the supernal Holy Trinity, and God created you and me to know, adore, and love God in His creation and Himself now and for eternity. Indeed, the best social and political order is the one that enables the most people possible to know *this* truth and practice it. It would be a fundamentally religious society—*truly* religious, that is, deeply spiritual and suffused with *agape,* not Pharisaical and cultish and full of hypocrisy and self-serving—founded upon and ordered to truth. Such a society would establish in positions of authority and power only those people and institutions most knowledgeable of and loving towards soul-enriching truths, beauties, and goods. And these leaders and institutions would seek to inculcate in the citizens through law and customs those virtues and practices that best enable such knowledge and love, virtues such as courage, temperance, justice, prudence, faith, hope, and love, and practices such as Socratic inquiry and dialectic, an economy of freedom, justice, charity, and leisure, and public celebrations and festivities that solidify the community in friendship and intensify our joy and solidarity by making explicit what and whom we love together.

How do contemporary societies and political orders measure up to our ideal society? Simone Weil's words above regarding her own society almost one hundred years before today are illuminating. With those with eyes to see, the evil now is so blatant and visceral, so profound and ubiquitous, so monstrous and ugly, so inhuman

and diabolical, it is akin to a Divine Revelation of evil. Murder and
lies are the trademarks of Satan, and the scamdemic is nothing but
murder, mass-global-genocidal murder, and lies, the greatest lies
ever uttered and practiced. Anyone who has plumbed the depth of
the evil of the scamdemic knows now, if he did not know before, that
money and power is not the purpose of life, that lying is evil, that
every human being is sacred, that God and love are real, and that
this world is wonderful and beautiful, but ultimately just a preparation for eternity, in comparison to which all created things are in-
substantial shadows. Here is the catechism of hell we were taught in
2020:

- Psychotic fear (as well as heart attacks and strokes in children) is normal.
- Official claims and pronouncements are always true, and arbitrary dictates, however cruel and irrational, must be
  obeyed without question.
- Healthy people are sick, indeed, are contagious and deadly
  walking diseases.
- The human face and breath are abominations to be covered
  and suffocated.
- Children should be tortured (mask-wearing for seven hours
  a day, even outside and when playing) and sacrificed (poison
  injections), even by their own mothers, for the comfort of
  adults.
- Universal and objective reality is off-limits to humanity, replaced by the declarations and dictates of self-and-state appointed "knowers."

Let us adapt Weil's words for our moment: So obvious are the *power and triumph of all men in the face of the plandemic*, which was supposed to be a machine only for breaking hearts and crushing spirits, a machine for manufacturing irresponsibility, stupidity, corruption, slackness and, above all, dizziness—*but has also, by God's grace, become a fountain of truth to embolden and enliven hearts, to empower responsibility, intelligence, purity, diligence, and above all, clarity.* For those with eyes and ears to see and hear, the Scamdemic was a revelation of pure evil, and so has revelatory, through contrast, of pure goodness. We know more than ever what goodness means and how important the truth is, for we have experienced their radical absence and negation. We are experiencing a worldwide *knowing* of truths that has been eclipsed and repressed for so many centuries due to the mass moral and spiritual lobotomization program that began in earnest in the "Enlightenment" and culminated in the postmodern dictatorship of relativism and technocratic totalitarian liberalism.[29] What do we know now?

- The human face is sacred and must never be shunned and covered as if it were intrinsically disgusting and evil and shameful.

---

[29] Michael Hanby, "The Birth of Liberal Order and the Death of God: A Reply to Robert Reilly's America on Trial — Part 1 of 3," *New Polity*, February 26, 2021, accessed December 17, 2024, https://newpolity.com/s/The-Birth-of-Liberal-Order-and-the-Death-of-God-Part-1.pdf.

- The simple things in life—good work, joyful play, wholesome parties, public fellowship in honest discussion and debate—these are precious and to be guarded with utmost vigilance from debilitating, suicidal fear and hatred.

- It is pure evil to wage power and submit to it when this power is not being used for the good, when it is arbitrary and disconnected from settled law and reality.

- There just *is* absolute Goodness, Truth, and Beauty, and our personal and social and economic and political life must be based upon these.

- We either have God and reality as the basis of our personal and corporate lives, or we have Satan and unreality.

- Liberalism, wherein the truth (except for "science") and the good (except for what's good for the oligarchs) are privatized and depoliticized, is an illusion. All political orders are predicated on, embody, and establish claims of truth and goodness.

Those most complicit in today's totalitarian evil desire hell on earth, but only as long as they get to rule over it. Those less complicit but still guilty of cowardice or greed or just apathy and passivity are okay with unreality and hell as long as they can have their little pleasures of judgment and scapegoating and their home-office tech jobs. But the rest of us want, more than ever before, reality and the heaven that is its essence, the reality/heaven that bespeaks and promises eternity and love and providence, the Fatherhood of God and the brotherhood of man under His loving protection and guidance. What we no longer want, after experiencing its hellish unreality for three years, is "the right to define one's own concept of existence, of meaning, of the universe, and of the mystery of human life," to use the words of Justice Anthony Kennedy in the *Planned Parenthood vs. Casey* Decision of 1992. For we know that this is not the "heart of liberty" as Kennedy assured us. At the heart of liberty is *reality*, God's reality, not the reality of technocratic eugenicists, sadistic billionaire psychopaths, soulless corporate and political puppets, and mindless, petty, and spiteful bureaucrats, and not even the reality as it appears to each of us in our inevitably ego-distorted consciousnesses. And we don't want a "concept of existence," either another's or our own, but existence itself. We don't want the right to *define* existence, but the ability to recognize, receive, adore, and love existence as it truly is.

Again, what we have experienced since the installation of liberalism in modernity is a slow process of moral, psychological, and spiritual retardation, where the masses have lost the ability to know and love the Good, satisfied with the simulacra of "defining" it by reducing it to shallow, propaganda-conditioned emotion and sheer, irrational, arbitrary will. And those who have managed to escape the dumbing-down process, who still retain the ability and desire to receive and love reality as it is, have been relegated to the margins of culture to live out their definitions and conceptions "of meaning, of the universe, and of the mystery of human life" in private social clubs.

Even after the unspeakable horrors of the World Wars, fascism, totalitarianism, genocides, IXXI, and the Global War of Terror, all of which were a sort of dry run for the more comprehensive and profound horrors we are now witnessing and to come, so many of us were still content with our postmodern bourgeoise lives of self-creation and our post-truth politics, as long as we had enough money and comfort and the freedom to live within our preferred sub-cultures. We took reality for granted, and our basic grasp of it, more or less accurately, we assumed with insouciance. And we didn't really care too much if our views of things *really* corresponded with reality, as long as they were "respectable" views. Even less did we care or even want politics to be based upon the actual Good and the morally and metaphysically and theologically True, but only on our contracted "rights" and "freedoms." If it secured those, to hell with reality, politically speaking. The Natural Law, the Tao, God's Will? Whatever. Politics can't be based on those now, with pluralism and freedom and all that. Most people are nice and leave you alone. We still have the power to vote and go to Church. Little did we know that in a few short years, reality itself would be taken from us and replaced with a counterfeit, a "concept of existence" of a few psychopaths imposed on the intimacies of our lives, with most of us embracing the counterfeit without hesitation and without even knowing it. D.C. Schinder articulates the pre-covid mindset:

> The absence of any social quality in truth leads to a peculiar dialectic in our relationship to our convictions. On the one hand, we affirm them with an odd detachment, a 'self-irony,' such as Vattimo advocates, and which may not even be conscious. We don't really believe anything. On the other hand, whatever attachment we do have becomes absolute, because it is unreflected and immediate, i.e., not mediated by reason.

In this respect, the conviction has the essential form of fanaticism, an emotional attachment that is immune to all reasoning. There is thus no incompatibility between half-hearted irony and fanatical conviction; these can reinforce each other, produce each other in an escalating way, turn immediately into each other, and even in some sense exist at once in the same mind. The tolerance that is expressly embraced as an ideal by the modern West therefore fosters at the same time an ethos of irrational violence. This ethos strangely increases at the very time that any apparent 'conflict' is neutralized; no one is denying you the right to hold it as true that leaves are green, and even to declare this publicly—under certain conditions: as long as, when you say, 'true,' you do not mean that anyone else would have any obligation to accept it against his arbitrary will.[30]

But this is all over. We are no longer ironic about our beliefs. And if we have a strong emotional and rigid conviction, it is not because we are fanatical but because we are grounded in reality. And we are indeed being denied the right to hold it as true that grass is green, but in this case, also these:

- That healthy people are healthy and not contagious, and sick people are sick and contagious.
- That masks do not protect you from a virus.

---

[30] David C. Schindler, *Love and the Postmodern Predicament: Rediscovering the Real in Beauty, Goodness, and Truth* (Grand Rapids, MI: Eerdmans, 2018), 18.

- That it is a form of mass torture to lock down the economy and mandate face-mask-wearing and social distancing of healthy people.
- That a "case" indicated by a medically non-diagnostic test doesn't mean you are sick or contagious with anything.
- That a casedemic is not a pandemic.
- That experimental, untested injections are dangerous, have shown to be injurious and fatal to many, and should never be mandated.
- That many people are still dropping dead in the streets—and athletic fields, and newsrooms, and in their sleep—and it's not from a virus.
- That there was no state of emergency due to "Covid-19," but one due to the bioweapon injections.
- That we are in a state of global totalitarianism based upon deliberate, malicious, and coordinated lies.
- That "the science" is a code word for propaganda.
- That virtually everyone in power is lying.

We are fighting to the death now for the right, not to define reality, but to reality itself. Pre-Covid, when, as good post-modern liberals, we lusted after the right to define reality for ourselves, we inadvertently gave that right to the most powerful, cruel, and ruthless, to corporations and states and media, and finally to the evilest human beings ever to live on God's green earth. And they proceeded to define reality for everyone else. Let us never go back to our vomit, but press on in the knowledge that God alone matters and God alone is Ultimate Reality. If we know this, we will love God and our neighbor, and heaven will come. Maranatha.

Are You Aware?

> The general public is being reduced to a state where people not only are unable to find about the truth but also become unable to search for the truth because they are satisfied with deception and trickery that have determined their convictions, satisfied with a fictitious reality created by design through the abuse of language.[31]

> Vision will blind.
> Severance ties.
> Median am I.
> True are all lies.[32]

There is a broad spectrum, as broad as the distance between heaven and hell, describing people's level of awareness of what is truly happening in the world today and why. The awareness abyss between those who know the truth and those who do not is a result of many things, including bad education and formation, a culture of lies, and the effect of the innumerable choices for or against reality

---

[31] Josef Pieper, "*Abuse of Language–Abuse of Power*" (San Francisco: Ignatius Press, 1992), 45.

[32] Meshuggah, "Sum," *Catch Thirty-three*, Nuclear Blast, 2005.

people have made in their lives, from the moment they became responsible for their choices, at the dawning of the age of reason, to the present moment. But the main reason for where people stand today vis-à-vis reality is the state of their souls vis-à-vis God. If I know and love God as a saint does, I will be aware of reality as it is; if I know and love God as a demon does, I will not be. And there are states in between.

Let me describe the awareness of someone on the lower side of the spectrum. There are myriad varieties of these people, depending on accidents of education, culture, socio-economic status, belief system, and political leanings. But at the core, the lack of awareness and alienation from reality is the same for all of them, and for the same essential reasons. I will begin with the most specific and superficial, in terms of geopolitical awareness, and end with the most general and profound spiritual awareness. I do not pretend to be at the highest level of awareness, but as Plato teaches us, when we truly leave one cave, we do know that we have left it, even if there are many more left to discover and from which to escape.

The low-level-awareness person thinks that there actually was a global pandemic and that it is, for all intents and purposes, over, as Biden has told them, thanks to the vaccine, the wise leadership of people like Tedros and Biden and Fauci and Gates, the heroic efforts of the best and brightest scientists and doctors, and the heroic sacrifices and selfless cooperation of the many good, responsible, loving citizens throughout the world. And it would have been over a long time ago if it weren't for Trump and the small number of his selfish, irresponsible, and disobedient followers, who, like spoiled children, wouldn't lockdown, "mask-up," and get the shot, and who believed in and promoted conspiracy theories that endangered public health and led to many deaths that could have been avoided. Biden said that they are an imminent and grave threat to our democracy, and he told the truth.

She thinks that in 2022 America began to defend Ukraine's freedom from Russia, being led by a new Hitler, and opposed by a courageous hero and new leader of the free world. She thinks that Ukraine was saved thanks to American assistance, just like in World War II when America rescued the Jews and the entire world from Hitler. She thinks that once Ukraine is liberated and Russia justly punished and chastised into submission (like Germany was), we can get back to the real and most formidable evil the world is facing, climate change. She is ready for all the sacrifices our leaders will ask us to make to bring about the final unification of the world under a global government, which will come about when divisive, racist, and outdated nations disappear. And just like with the pandemic, we will vanquish this great evil of nationhood that our unenlightened predecessors bequeathed to us, which is the final obstacle preventing us from establishing a new world order of peace and prosperity and happiness for all. Oh, and the high gas and food prices? Those will go away soon, she assures us, just as soon as the MAGA people are eradicated, Putin is assassinated, and everyone gets their 18th booster. Sit tight, be patient, and get used to much less white privilege. Eating bugs isn't that bad. Less calories.

He sees the overturning of Roe vs. Wade in 2022 as only a temporary setback in the ongoing and inexorable struggle for individual freedom and women's rights, whose victory is assured and imminent, as witnessed by the exponential increase in freedom over the last decade, with the right to gender-reassignment surgery for children being only the latest triumph among many more to come. He awaits eagerly the new technological advances that will, like contraception and abortion pills, mRNA vaccines, and the Metaverse, enable humans to further evolve into full adulthood and take control over that evolution, so that the last vestiges of our imprisoning givenness can be sloughed off and we can finally become the kind of beings that for far too long we projected onto gods and God due to the ignorance, self-hatred, and cowardice of our religious forebears. He loves what he sees in Pope Francis, and especially the German Synod, because he is taking the Catholic Church in the right direction of diversity and inclusion, although it has a lot of catching up to do.

Why these views? For the answer, we must move from a description of these persons' low-level, reality-averse awareness of what is happening socially, culturally, and politically to their even lower-level awareness of historical, metaphysical, and moral reality from which they derive their asinine opinions. The following is one version of their historical narrative, translated into the highfalutin English of the typical idiotic academic:

Only in secular modernity did man finally achieve his liberation from oppression and ignorance, from superstition, magic, tyranny, and priestcraft, from the dark forces of religious power, fanatical belief, and sectarianism. Man achieved this liberation primarily through the secularization of reason, morality and society, which included the separation of religion from the political order, the church from the

state. Ever-increasing religious and ideological pluralism ensued as soon as men of good will were permitted to exercise
freely their reason and act on their consciences. It is certainly
the case that when Christendom was finally broken up in the
wake of the Reformation, religiously intolerant, confessional, monarchical states emerged, but these evolved quite
quickly, historically speaking, into the secular, tolerant, pluralistic, democratic states we have today. The rise of secular
society after the sixteenth and seventeenth-century wars of
religion was rendered possible only by the removal of religion from all positions of political significance and power.
Good-willed, reasonable people were ready and willing to accept the desacralization of the state after decades of incessant
bloodshed over religion. Sequestered, depoliticized, and privatized, religion and the sacred would now no longer cause
war, divisiveness, and oppression, and the newly liberated,
autonomous, politically secular individual could finally
thrive. In the religiously tolerant, secular, pluralistic liberal
democracy governed by the rights of men, not God, the sacred would still have a place and a capacity to exert influence
over politics, but now it would have to coexist with the many
competing sacreds residing in the same city, proliferating
and dwelling together in peace precisely because none are
permitted to obtain societal, cultural, and political power, let
alone a monopoly on power. In short, secular modernity was
born when the archaic, violence-inducing sacred lost its public, political hegemony and influence, being relegated to the
sub-political, private sphere of men's fancies and hearts.

What took its place in the public square is what should have always been there in the first place, the right of individuals to self-determination, to freedom of thought, action, speech, and religion. In modernity man had the courage and intelligence to attempt, for the first time in human history, to construct a political order not based upon the religious, the sacred. While not denying the right of every citizen to believe in a sacred, superhuman, cosmic, divine, transcendent power as the true ground of man's existence, both personal and social, the theoreticians of the modern paradigm, people such as Machiavelli, Hobbes, Locke, Rousseau, Kant, and Madison, decided that secular values and rights, codified in a social contract, would replace any supposed power or will higher than man. And we are so thankful they did.

Such are these persons' core metaphysical beliefs: Mindless matter is all there is, well, except for *my* Mind, which is free and limitless, though determined by economics—but I'm free. I am a free spirit, though there are no spirits. And truth is the opinion of the powerful, which is oppressive and untrue, unless I'm in power; or perhaps it's the opinion of the marginalized. And all opinions are equal, except those that aren't, like Science and Critical Race Theory. And as for morality—it's relative, period. Except for racism and sexism and homophobia, which are absolute evils. And MAGA is evil. But good and evil are the labels of the intolerant, or the rationalizations of class consciousness, but vaccines are absolutely good and people should be forced to get them, and Putin is evil. And we today in the 21st century are morally superior to everyone who lived before us, except that we're all equal. And abortion is good, so it should be imposed on everyone, but morality is relative. Freedom is the Good, and the Good is Freedom—except for the freedom to try to make something other than freedom the Good, which must be stopped, by force if need be. Spiritually, these persons believe in love, or power, or both, or nothing. The diversity of religions is willed by God, except those religions that claim to be the true religion, which God, who doesn't exist because we are God, hates. Jesus was a nice man and a good moral teacher, but some of his disciples were anti-semitic, such as St. John and St. Paul. Crusades. Inquisition. Nazism. Trump. We know all this now and have sought or demanded forgiveness and groveling, and that's why we love Pope Francis. The universal religion of love is sweeping across the planet, as we await its definitive spokesperson. It is already showing itself, as evidenced by divinely inspired masterpieces of art like this one:

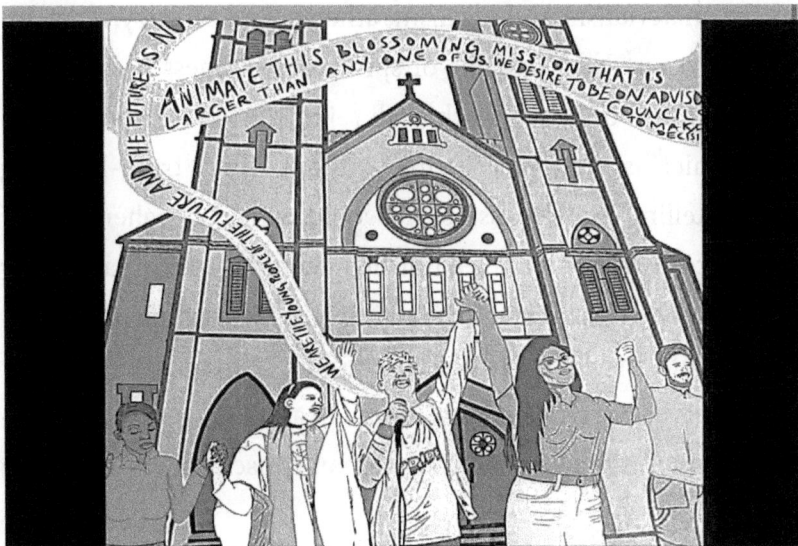

The lockdowns were the first fruits of the New Spirit, bringing us all together in sacrificial love and Science. And the Vaccine is our new sacrament:

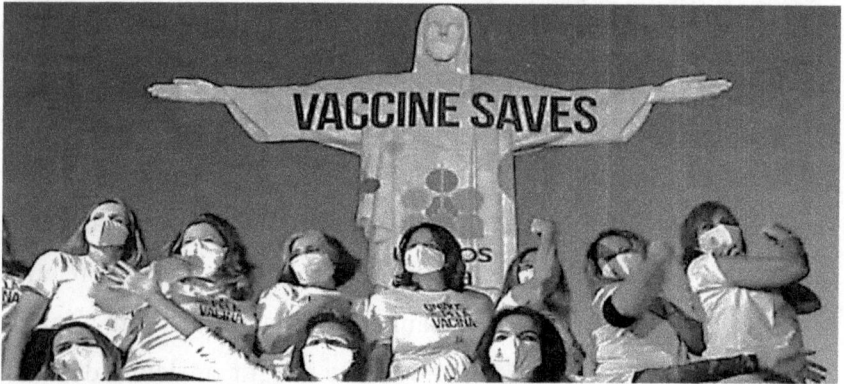

The moral, metaphysical, and spiritual beliefs of the low-level awareness people are, of course, incoherent, a mishmash of relativism, absolutism, particularism, universalism, self-righteousness and self-deprecation, individualism and collectivism, nihilism and crusaderism, materialism and idealism, atheism and idolatry. They indicate the lowest level possible of spiritual awareness because, despite the illusion of diversity, they all reject the law of non-contradiction, which is the first principle without which truth-knowing and truth-telling are impossible. It would evince a higher level of metaphysical awareness to be a full-fledged materialist or atheist or nihilist, for at least there would be an implicit recognition of the possibility of truth, even if the truth claim itself is self-contradictory and false. But this eclectic spirituality, rooted in a chaotic moral and metaphysical soup, is the very nadir of human consciousness and is the perfect breeding ground for global totalitarianism and the Antichrist who will soon embody it and impersonate it, literally.

Why would someone holding this set of moral, metaphysical, and spiritual attitudes or moods—let us not dignify them with the word *beliefs*—endorse the forced covering of one's face and injections into one's body, the placing of the entire world under house arrest, the censoring of all speech not in line with arbitrary "expert" claims, the requiring of papers to be live society, the greatest wealth transfer in history to the richest elites on the planet, a NATO war of aggression against a nuclear power and a Zionist genocide, on the one hand, and the genital mutilation and sexualization of children, murdering babies, sodomy, and cannibalism (coming soon), and the replacement of popular entertainment with satanic occult rituals, on the other? It is because the upshot of those "beliefs" is the promise of power to their adherents, for they are all predicated on the rejection of any authority above man's will. And since the collective will always trumps the individual one due to the dynamic of sheer power, which is all that is left when there is nothing above the human will; since the most powerful and ruthless elites always dominate the collective will; and since Satan always dominates the most powerful and ruthless, the will of Satan will be done on earth as it is in Hell when the conditions are ripest for his enthronement. Those conditions exist perfectly among the lowest-level awareness people, and to only a slightly lesser extent among those of higher-level awareness, which, apart from the very highest, is still very, very low. It is only those with the very highest-level awareness who stand in the way of the coming of the Antichrist at this time, and will recognize him when he comes.

What are the geopolitical, moral, metaphysical, and spiritual beliefs of those with this highest level of awareness? Well, I wish I knew them, and to say that I do is to arrogantly imply that I am among these. I daresay that I try to follow those institutions, traditions, and personages that have proven their exquisite level of awareness through their works and fruits, their holiness, integrity, courage, charity, and prophetic witness. Suffice it to say, I try to know, love, and obey reality, a sign of a high-level awareness in an Age of Unreality. What is this reality according to these authorities?

For geopolitical reality, if it is true that we are in a state of full-fledged global totalitarianism, and to see this one must already have a high level of awareness, then those institutions and people telling the full truth would be infallibly detected by the vehemence of the attacks against them by the Global Regime of Lies. The highest level of awareness, then, can be described accurately and simply by compiling the claims of these. No institution is attacked more frequently, ferociously, and insidiously than the Catholic Church, both from without and within, both by intimidation and persecution, seduction and infiltration. Therefore, just read the Catechism of the Catholic Church for an infallible description of the highest level of awareness in terms of moral, metaphysical, and spiritual truth.

In terms of historical narrative, the highest level of awareness can thus be found by rejecting any political history that denigrates the Catholic Church and rejects its true reality as the Mystical Body of Christ, and that doesn't see the Incarnation as the center of human history. For example, awareness knows that the City of God is founded on a love of God that leads its citizens to contempt for themselves, counting all earthly things as worthless. St. Augustine argues that the temporal ought to be ordered to the eternal, but that this ordering will never be achieved until the second coming of the Lord. For, there is a second city here on earth in addition to the city of God— the *civitas terrena*, the earthly city. This city is founded on a love of self to the contempt of God. And these two cities are in conflict. The earthly city is always opposed to true religion. Justice consists in giving each his own, thus no society is just that does not give God the worship due to Him.

The following narrative of liberal democracy and the so-called Enlightenment is the high-awareness counterpoint to the low-awareness narrative described above, and anyone holding anything like this narrative would be immediately fired from any mainstream academic or government position. Since the Fall, man has attempted to flee the ubiquitous reality of God through creative abstraction from the natural things of His creation and the supernatural plan of His redemption. Fallen man has always been offended at the "scandal of particularity," always seeking to live in a universe of his own devising, always abstracting from the concrete, contingent, fleshy, historical realities in which he, as a creature of matter and spirit, finds himself, and through which God has chosen to communicate Himself to him. All was well in the Garden until Adam and Eve began abstracting: "It can't be this particular fruit on this particular tree that could be so significant to God and to our happiness!" For the ancient Greek philosophers, God's existence was knowable; for the Jews, He was a living presence. But that he would limit Himself to a backwater village in the Middle East, or become anything less than a divine conqueror, was foolishness to the former and a stumbling block to the latter. Martin Luther accepted the truth that the universal became particular in the Incarnation, but denied that this Incarnation should be seen as continuing mystically in a particular, historical, visible institution demanding man's obedience. Enlightenment man accepted the existence of God and absolute truth, but demanded that these be universally accessible solely through man's reason. "Enlightenment" would be the result of abstracting from one's particular and contingent cultural and religious "superstitions" to attain the universal truth transcending them. But such a position was tantamount to abstracting the Incarnation out of reality, to rejecting the entire supernatural order made manifest in and through Our Lord, and denying the necessity of His grace and teachings for an accurate understanding and practice of even natural truth and virtue. Postmodern man appeared to have overcome this error, rightly rejecting Enlightenment man's facile claim to have discovered self-evident absolute truths in abstraction from particularist commitments. He discovered that the historical, the cultural, the societal, that is, the particular, cannot be so easily cut out of the picture. "Self-evident"—to whom? A fair question, that.

Yet by denying the possibility of attaining universal truth through and in its particular embodiments, the atheist-oriented postmodernists rejected the reality of transcendence for the abstraction of pure immanence. In short, every error of man throughout history has been the result of missing the balance between immanence and transcendence, the human and the divine, the particular and the universal, by abstracting out some realm of natural or supernatural reality. The diabolically fomented World Wars of our past century, the plandemic, and the WWIII we are now in sapped the life out of the religious and cultural tradition of the West, with the anti-traditional abstractions of communism, fascism, Nazism, neo-liberalism, and the Great Reset serving as demonic parodies of the Catholic Church. But Lucifer's coup de grâce would be saved for our century. To his dismay, his all-out destructive assault on tradition in the first half of the twentieth century had provoked a robust counterattack by men of goodwill in the second half. Lucifer learned his lesson: men cannot exist without some sort of tradition. Thus, instead of attempting again the direct destruction of the Western Christian tradition (rendered rather vestigial, decrepit, and paltry, it must be admitted, from his first assault), this time he pursued a subtler but more effective method. Realizing that any authentic tradition, even a barely breathing one, is a receiver and transmitter of the divine, his stroke of genius was to inspire the construction and establishment of an abstract anti-tradition that would receive and transmit nothing. Although similar in its unreality to the abstractions of communism, fascism, Nazism, and globalism, it would bear such a striking resemblance to the Christian tradition that it would escape detection. Implemented surreptitiously and cloaking itself in the form of its host, it would serve as the tradition to end all tradition. Not only would there be no counterattack this time, men of good will would have no idea what hit them—or even that they had been hit.

Secular liberal democracy is the cave, liberalism the shadows on its walls, and "conservative," "liberal," and "radical" shadows of various shapes and sizes. For those in the cave, reality is contacted by comparing and choosing among the shadows; certain shadows appear "true," while other shadows seem "false." But since shadows are all they know, it cannot be said that they really know any of these shadows at all. They do not know the shadows as shadows. They may use the word "shadow" in their many echoey, cave discussions, but they do not know of what the shadows are shadows. Indeed, if they ever recognized the shadows as shadows, they would escape the cave. Liberalism is just such a cave. People in the modern West may use the term "liberalism," and identify "other" points of view in contrast to it, but because they are inside liberalism and do not know it, they do not recognize the liberalism of liberalism. They do not see it as an alien, artificial ideology projected upon the walls of their minds by the elitist puppeteers of academia, religion, bureaucracy, and media, but simply as "just the way things are." They are like fish that never recognize their immersion in water because they know of nothing else.

Liberalism claims to provide a religiously neutral social framework within which individuals can autonomously determine their own vision of the world in perfect freedom. But we must reject liberalism's official public claim that it lacks any particular conception of the good and any restrictions on others' conceptions of the good. Since liberal culture is founded upon a particular conception of the good and a particular doctrine of truth—namely, the good of the privatization of all claims to truth, and the truth of the irreducible plurality of conceptions of the good—and since the publicly authoritative rhetoric of liberal culture denies having any substantive conceptions of its own, what liberalism amounts to is an established and intolerant belief system—a religion—that indoctrinates citizens into disbelieving in its very existence. Just as the puppeteers must ensure that the shadows are never recognized as shadows, lest the cave be identified as a cave and the prisoners break their chains; liberalism must never be exposed as liberalism, that is, as a historically contingent, non-necessary, manmade ideology. It must at all costs be identified with "the facts," "the way things are," as the inexorable social reality. In short, as the great Nietzschean ironist Stanley Fish, a cave puppeteer with a genius for exposing his fellow puppeteers to the light, has confessed: "liberalism doesn't exist."[33]

The problem, however, is that it does, and its existence is no longer limited to an abstract idea or a revolutionary experiment—it is now a well-established social reality. The liberal incubus has found a willing consort in the decrepit culture of the secularized West, and unfortunately, we citizens of the modern liberal democracies of the West are its traditionalists. Cavanaugh's name for liberalism is the "worship of the empty shrine":

> The public shrine has been emptied of any one particular God or creed, so that the government can never claim divine sanction and each person may be free to worship as she sees fit.... There is no single visible idol, no golden calf, to make the idolatry obvious . . . officially the shrine remains empty.... The empty shrine, however, threatens to make a deity not out of God but out of our freedom to worship God. Our freedom comes to occupy the empty shrine. Worship becomes worship of our collective self, and civil religion tends to marginalize the worship of the true God.[34]

---

[33] See Stanley Fish, "Mission Impossible: Settling the Just Bounds Between Church and State," *Columbia Law Review* 97, no. 8 (1997): 2255–2333.

[34] William T. Cavanaugh, *Migrations of the Holy: God, State, and the Political*

With a track record of human sacrifice, how has the empty shrine of liberal nothing-worship (to conflate names for a moment) managed to escape our detection? The short answer is that it has removed our eyes. Authentic traditions, both natural and supernatural, embody and transmit the ultimate realities of man's existence, the transcendent origin, end, and meaning of things that cannot be grasped by the isolated individual, and cannot be fully rationalized or defined.

Ultimate reality must be experienced through and in its incarnation in tradition. It is in this sense that tradition is the eye that allows men to see the spiritual, eternal, and transcendent meanings hidden in the physical, temporal, and mundane facts of everyday existence. Participants in the anti-tradition of liberalism, however, are prevented from ever seeing themselves as participants in a tradition, even though they are its slaves. They are blinded to their God-given identity as members of a common good higher than themselves, even as they serve as mere cogs in the liberal machine. The freedom cult includes all others, even the cult of the Eucharist, and so it is more universal, more "catholic," and therefore more divine than the Eucharist. By not prescribing any particular object of public devotion, the State's empty shrine appears to allow all devotions to exist and thrive more successfully than if there were an exclusivist, established cult, such as Catholicism. However, all of this is a grand illusion. As David Schindler points out: "The state cannot finally avoid

Meaning of the Church (Grand Rapids, MI: Wm. B. Eerdmans Publishing Co., 2011), 123.

affirming, in the matter of religion, a priority of either 'freedom from' or 'freedom for'—both of these imply a theology."[35]

In the end, we are each responsible for our level of awareness, and God created us to aspire to the highest level possible, the intimate awareness of Him. We can only become aware of our unawareness by His grace, and we need His minute-by-minute help to ascend to higher and higher levels, lest we fall backward into our own darkness and blindness. Let us practice the presence of God always so that we become more and more aware of His indescribable love for us and share this awareness with all whom we meet.

Will Anyone Resist the Antichrist when He Comes?

And we beseech you, brethren, by the coming of our Lord Jesus Christ, and of our gathering together unto him, that you be not easily moved from your sense, nor be terrified, neither by spirit, nor by word, nor by epistle, as sent from us, as if the day of the Lord were at hand. Let no man deceive you by any means, for unless there come a revolt first, and the man of sin be revealed, the son of perdition, who opposeth and is lifted up above all that is called God or that is worshipped, so that he sitteth in the temple of God, shewing himself as if he were God. Remember you not that when I was yet with you I told you these things?

---

[35] David L. Schindler, *The Heart of the World, the Center of the Church: Communio Ecclesiology, Liberalism, and Liberation* (Grand Rapids, MI: Wm. B. Eerdmans Publishing Co., 1996), 184

And now you know what withholdeth, that he may be revealed in his time. For the mystery of iniquity already worketh; only that he who now holdeth do hold until he be taken out of the way. And then that wicked one shall be revealed whom the Lord Jesus shall kill with the spirit of his mouth and shall destroy with the brightness of his coming, him whose coming is according to the working of Satan, in all power and signs and lying wonders, and in all seduction of iniquity to them that perish; because they receive not the love of the truth that they might be saved. Therefore God shall send them the operation of error to believe lying, that all may be judged who have not believed the truth but have consented to iniquity. But we ought to give thanks to God always for you, brethren beloved of God, for that God hath chosen you first fruits unto salvation in sanctification of the spirit and faith of the truth.[36]

Dr. Peter Hotez is the Bill Nye the Science Guy of Vaccines, bow-tie and all. Anyone with any position of public prominence in vaccines, whether a Big Pharma executive or local doctor, and who has endorsed them, is either materially (unknowingly) or formally (knowingly) complicit in mass murder. For Hotez, it is undoubtedly formal complicity, for he is an obvious liar and fraud and grifter. He's an insider, so he knows the vax is a deadly bioweapon, and he promotes it—religiously—anyway, either because he likes that millions of people are being murdered by it, or he likes the money and

---

[36] *The Holy Bible: Douay-Rheims Version* (Charlotte, NC: Saint Benedict Press, 2009), 2 Thess. 2:1-12.

prestige he is getting for promoting it, or both. It's hard to tell which option is correct. Most recently, he "warned" Americans that multiple viruses could strike America right after Trump takes office in January of 2025.[37] If that sounds less like a warning than a threat, it's because it is. This guy is pure evil.

He has been challenged to debate RFK, Jr., who was appointed by President Trump to be the Secretary of the Department of Health and Human Services in November of 2024, and he was offered 2.7 million dollars to do it. He refused the challenge and, of course, he will never do it. The reason is that such a debate would actually be about the truth, and not just rhetorical spin and manipulation, and would thus lead to some truth being revealed to the public in a public way. And since the main goal of a totalitarian regime, of which Hotez is a top commissar, is to murder the authority of truth and replace it with power, its diabolical counterfeit, a public debate with RFK, Jr., a truth teller about vaccines (though not about abortion and Israel), would be, let's say, counterproductive.

Has the totalitarianism of the past four years reached its goal of murdering the authority of truth? It has, I think, to a large extent, both in the world and in the Church. This murder campaign has been underway since the rebellion of Lucifer and the Fall of Man, but Jesus reestablished the authority of Truth by His Incarnation, Crucifixion, and Resurrection; the Holy Spirit institutionalized it throughout the world in the Church, Christ's Bride, of which the

---

[37] Srishti B Dutta, "Vaccine Researcher Peter Hotez Warns Multiple Viruses Could Strike America Right after Trump Takes Office," India Times, December 25, 2024, https://www.indiatimes.com/trending/social-relevance/vaccine-researcher-peter-hotez-warns-multiple-viruses-could-strike-america-right-after-trump-takes-office-647601.html.

Holy Spirit is her soul; and Christendom created a civilization founded on widespread corporate obedience to this authority, suppressing the power-worshiping pagan system of sorcery and scapegoating. But the forces of evil destroyed Christendom, and the Church hierarchy today, and way too many of the laity, has all but internalized the commands of her oppressors. It looks to me that in March 2020, the *katechon* was removed, and so the appearance of the *anomos*, the man of lawlessness, is imminent. Indeed, the reign of lawlessness has already appeared, with its millions of subjects in both high and low places committing an ever-increasing amount, in both quantity and depravity, of crimes against God and men constituting a coordinated summoning incantation in a liturgy of evil to culminate in the manifestation of its King.

The first law to be rejected in this black mass is the law of truth, which commands us always to place truth above all other desires or considerations. The rejection of truth, then, precedes and causes all other forms of lawlessness. "Do what thy will shall be the whole of the law," the first commandment of Satanism, is the rejection of truth and its replacement with power. Here is an excellent description by "The Ethical Skeptic" of the typical traits of these truthless men who image and are now summoning their father, Antichrist:

> They enjoy or are addicted to the loosh derived from witnessing or inflicting pain in others. Their first instinct is to seek symbolism, authority, dominance, final disposition, or control. They are quickly threatened by competence (watch for this discomfort flag when you read a room). Every act is

a manipulation towards an end/nothing is derived from objective neutrality. They conceal their inner nature/put on an identity of virtue (the opposite of ethics). They will habitually misrepresent what you say, often just to see if you will catch the straw man. They do not actually engage to discuss the topic at hand, their focus quickly and habitually gravitates to you. Every utterance is an attack or a premise to one. Every thought features a weaponized buzzword of some sort. The Narrative is their habitual fortress of correctness, from which they cowardly scorn others. Anyone who disagrees with them fits neatly into buckets of habitual derision. They will obsess over made up *quo facto malo* offenses their victims have 'committed'. Everyone they harm is a 'narcissist', for saying, doing, or being something without their permission. Their complete absence of any reference to self betrays an enormous conceit. They leave you with an uncomfortable dank feeling. They find joy in making people look or feel stupid, it is a drug they desperately seek. If an observer recounts an observation, they will comment upon the aspect of it which portrays the observer in the most negative light, as opposed to most positive light, or the observation itself. They show no remorse nor respect for boundaries. They find the young and vulnerable, exciting. Their logic is rife with *auto-aufheben* appeal wherein one statement will falsify their next. They are penny wise and pound foolish in all matters of discernment aside from greed. They find entertainment in highlighting other's errors or insulting them. They don't take responsibility for nor recall their own actions. Deaths, virtue, justice, science, climate, pandemic, racism, migration, poverty – these are all cudgels as opposed to stemming from a heartfelt mercy. They are 'non-violent' as long as they cannot get away with violence. They mock the misfortune of others. Their few friends, don't really know them and are exactly like them. They are/were once cruel to animals or had 'psychological issues'. They derive great joy in the authoritative cleverness of a lie, the larger and more intimidating the lie, the better. They fail to associate their poor state in life with their dark habits. They don't bear an ability to introspect. Aside from memorized pablum, they don't really get philosophy/ethics. Your disagreement at their condemnation of you, is further evidence of your guilt. Even though they constantly fixate or maintain the focus upon others, everything is in fact about them.[38]

Now, it is true that these traits characterize the malignant narcissist or the textbook psychopath. Still, it seems to me that more and more ordinary people are displaying these traits, a sort of acquired psychopathy due to immersion in our totalitarian anti-truth culture.

It is the ultimate irony that "the science" has replaced "the truth" in public discourse, though ostensibly conveying the same meaning, namely, that which transcends mere opinion because justified by an evidential appeal to what is the case in reality. For it is now nothing

---

[38] The Ethical Skeptic, "How to Detect a Griefer," October 15, 2020, https://theethicalskeptic.com/2020/10/15/how-to-detect-a-griefer/.

but the opinion of the strongest, meaning those who control the supply of money and levers of power, and hence what opinions have authority in public discourse. Those who condemn this corruption of the Word are, tellingly, ridiculed as "truthers." In other words, those who insist that reality itself, what is actually good, be the standard for the coercive use of power, and not the naked, arbitrary will of the powerful—such as the will of school district superintendents to show pornography to Kindergarten children—are now considered evil or mentally deranged (in spite of the fact that the definition of a crazy person is someone not in touch with reality), a "domestic terror" threat.

It makes sense why a narcissist or psychopath would be indifferent to the authority of truth, for he is, as inexplicable as this is, incapable of obeying it—he is a literal slave to his desires. And it is understandable why your everyday wicked person, one who has willfully and consistently chosen to do evil by making money or power or prestige his God over goodness and reality, would defy the authority of truth, for he knows he is supposed to obey reality, but for whatever reason would rather have the lower objects of their desires than that which actually makes them happy. But what we are dealing with today makes no sense: ordinary non-psychopaths and non-wicked people for whom truth is simply not a concern, let alone an authority.

All that matters to these new "men without chests"[39] is whether their feelings, opinions, and actions conform to what they consider to be the "right" feelings, opinions, and actions, with *right* having

---

[39] See C.S Lewis, *The Abolition of Man* (Oxford: Oxford University Press, 1943).

nothing to do with being in accord with goodness or reality, but only with an identity in a narrative wherein they are superior to others. Whether this narrative is true or not is not even a consideration. Indeed, if asked, they would insist that there are no *true* narratives, or beliefs, for belief in the truth of some beliefs and not others is exclusive and intolerant and arrogant and supremacist, etc.—it doesn't fit with their identity as the superior ones. What makes them superior is simply believing in and parroting the narrative, and what makes them believe in and parrot the narrative is simply that it is what superior people do.

One can be confident that the Antichrist, the man of lawlessness, is soon to appear on the world stage because the people who will follow him, which is to say, nearly everyone in the Western world and those outside the West who have been habituated into its diabolical existential orientation, have already been doing so for some time in their treasonous attitude towards Truth. The Antichrist's religion, a global and totalitarian, spiritual stranglehold that will absorb every aspect of life, politics, economics, culture, health, science, education, etc., will make no truth claims, yet demand full adherence of intellect, heart, and will to its dogmas and commands. To be one of its practitioners will require no virtue and goodness of will, but all its members will be convinced of their virtue and goodness and the evil of all non-members, you know, the haters, conspiracy theorists, white supremacists, and domestic terrorists. To imagine what this religion might look like in practice, just take the phenomenon we witnessed from 2020-2023 of mothers forcing their small children to wear suffocating masks for hours on end, taking them to the "doctor" to receive deadly bioweapon injections, and bringing them to libraries to be entertained by grown men thrusting their groins into their faces. Now, take the fact of these otherwise unimaginable and unspeakable evils (they were unimaginable and unspeakable only four years ago), add to it that these mothers and the society at large deem this behavior loving and virtuous and "progressive"—what the superior people do—and then realize that what we are witnessing today is just a small prelude to and mere hint of the behavior that the Antichrist religion will require and which will become the standard of goodness and virtue when it is finally established in the world.

To be accepted into the Antichrist's religion, with all the worldly rewards that this will bring, will only really require one thing—that you believe in it with your whole heart, mind, and strength. because, and only because, it is *untrue*. To believe in something because it is true, not because it is "correct," and to do something because it is good, not because it is what superior people do, is already, to a certain extent, to worship God, because it implies acceptance of and obedience to the authority of Reality, even if one gets reality wrong due to miseducation or a passion-compromised conscience. Our culture is already well on its way to making it all but impossible for people to accept, let alone obey, the authority of Truth. Add to it the irresistible rewards (financial, social, political, psychological, emotional, "spiritual") that will come instantly to anyone who renounces Truth once and for all, and finally, the onslaught of a ubiquitous and irresistible, hurricane-lie contagion of scapegoating directed at those who don't, and it is reasonable to surmise that when Antichrist arrives, for all those who have been cooperating in the last few years with the pandemic of treason against Truth, he will be impossible to resist.

Chapter II

The War

Freedom vs God

Distrust, fear
Separation is the division that binds us
Broken minds in a distorted world, out of balance
Incongruous and tenuous
The fear that permeates this world is a sickness
A plight on mankind, a blight to our world
This monstrosity of creation moves forth
Earth constantly threatens
Age constantly beckons
The looming is beyond tangible[1]

When the fear and hysteria, mask mandates, and lockdowns began in March of 2020, I knew that massive and coordinated political power was being used for great evil. I also knew, somehow, that the main purpose of it was to coerce the masses into getting a poisonous injection. My response was to try to stop the evil, through speaking, writing, and activism. The activist groups I created and joined, both physical and digital, all had the name "freedom" in them, as if to imply that the goal was to return a political power gone totalitarian

---

[1] Krallice, "Kronos Deposed," on *Loüm*, released October 27, 2017, streaming audio.

to its proper scope and authority, to promote and secure freedom. By this, they clearly meant a certain legally protected, unpoliced space of individual and group activity free from all coercive pressure and intervention, whether by the state or by other citizens. Of course, the plandemic spokesmen assured us that this was all just a temporary and exceptional use of coercive political power in order to secure individual freedom in the long run. But in the short run—fifteen days to stop the spread—what was necessary was decisive collective action involving temporary restrictions of individual freedom and otherwise freely exercised rights. The clear implication was that in exceptional circumstances, the "common good" requires personal sacrifice, and in this case, since the sacrifices needed to be immediate, specific, and highly coordinated, and only the medical experts knew the right protocol, what would otherwise have been purely voluntary sacrifices had to be coercively mandated. The logic of this seemed airtight and reasonable, so the vast majority complied, assuring themselves that the freedoms to which they were entitled and accustomed would soon be returned.

It has been over four years of totalitarian hell, and other than a few insignificant wins for individual freedom and rights, what the totalitarians took away they have not given back. They have loosened the pandemic screws a bit, but they can tighten them at any time, or create new and larger screws through another global psy-op trauma event. As I write this, there is talk of a "bird flu" and coming lockdowns. And no amount of protest from the relatively few anti-totalitarians who managed not to internalize the commands of our

oppressors will, it seems, be able to stop them. The woke totalitarianism is now in full swing, and the anti-woke seem helpless to stop
this satanic juggernaut. It just has too much power.

The evil that has entrenched itself at the very center and heart of
political and cultural power not only purports to have authority over
us but also, it seems, actually possesses it. It is as if it had a *right* to
be there, and a metaphysical or spiritual *right*, not a merely human
or legal one. Exorcists tell us that the exorcism only works when it
can reveal the legal right the demon has somehow obtained to possess its victim, for only then can it undo this legal contract, whether
created by the curse of another or the voluntary invitation of the victim, through the exorcism prayers and the renunciation and repentance of the victim. My point is that the demon actually has a God-
given right to the power he exercises, and nothing but the undoing
of the right can vanquish it. To do this, the victim must renounce his
idolatry, for all sin is a form of idolatry, putting some creature in the
place of God in the soul, and then worship, explicitly and intention-
ally, Jesus Christ. Notice that the demon will only leave when the
victim both renounces Satan *and* surrenders to Jesus Christ. The
soul cannot remain neutral. I think that the demon that is now pos-
sessing the ruling elite, and through them, the collective soul of
America, as well as the West as a whole (and the East, to a certain
extent), has a right to be there, as a product of both a curse and a
voluntary invitation. The Christian West in general and the Catholic
Church in particular were cursed a long time ago by high-ranking
Freemasons. But we also invited the demon in.

When a person refuses to worship the Living God, he doesn't
stop worshipping, for we are worshipping animals by nature. He

may think he is agnostic or pluralist, or religiously neutral, but this is just verbal obfuscation. There is always some, single, overarching object of desire around which one's life is oriented and to which all one's thoughts, words, desires, and actions are ordered and submitted, one ultimate authority to which one gives his obedience—even if this authority is not clearly recognized or understood. It's there in the background, nevertheless. And if this object of desire and ruling authority is not God, the True God revealed in and as Jesus Christ, it will be some kind of idol. And when there is idol worship, there is sin, and thus an open invitation to demonic influence, including the possibility of demonic possession. Such is the same for societies and political communities.

"And he said to them, 'Go into all the world and proclaim the good news to the whole creation. The one who believes and is baptized will be saved; but the one who does not believe will be condemned.'"[2] This proclamation and the consequences for its acceptance or rejection by individual persons also applies to nations, as man is a political animal, as *Dignitatis humanae*, the *Declaration on Religious Liberty* of Vatican II, makes clear: "Religious freedom, in turn, which men demand as necessary to fulfill their duty to worship God, has to do with immunity from coercion in civil society. Therefore it leaves untouched traditional Catholic doctrine on the moral duty of individuals and societies toward the true religion and toward the one Church of Christ."[3]

---

[2] Mark 16:15–16 (NRSV).

[3] Second Vatican Council. *Dignitatis Humanae* (Declaration on Religious Freedom), December 7, 1965, no. 1. https://www.vatican.va/archive/hist_councils/ii_vatican_council/documents/vat-ii_decl_19651207_dignitatis-humanae_en.html.

Why do societies have this duty to worship God? Here is Cardinal Alfredo Ottaviani, from the preliminary document for the Second Vatican Council, "On the Relations Between the Church and the State and On Religious Tolerance":

The civil authority cannot be indifferent with regard to religion. Instituted by God in order to help men acquire a truly human perfection, it must not only supply its subjects with the possibility of procuring temporal goods for themselves, either material or intellectual, but besides favor the abundance of spiritual goods, permitting people to lead a human life in a religious manner. Now, among these goods, nothing is more important than to know and to recognize God, and then to fulfill one's duties towards God: here indeed is the foundation of all private and, still more, public virtue. These duties towards God oblige, towards the divine Majesty, not only each one of the citizens but also the civil authority, which, in its public acts, incarnates civil society. God is indeed the author of civil society and the source of all the goods which flow down through it to its members. Civil society must therefore honor and serve God. As for the manner of serving God, this can be no other, in the present economy, than that which He Himself has determined, as obligatory, in the true Church of Christ; and this not only in the person of the citizens, but equally in that of the Authorities who represent civil society.[4]

---

[4] Central Pontifical Commission Preparatory to the Second Vatican Council,

Now, it is true, of course, that when the majority population of a nation is not Catholic, there can be no just establishment of the Catholic Church as the spiritual authority over the people, for, as Ottaviani makes clear, "the civil authority is not permitted in any way to compel consciences to accept the Faith revealed by God. Indeed, the Faith is essentially free and cannot be the object of any constraint, as the Church teaches by saying, 'That no one be compelled to embrace the Catholic Faith unwillingly.'" Nevertheless, this does not entail that political authority can be neutral towards God or religion, let alone the moral law. It must promote the truth insofar as it is known by reason, which includes some foundational religious truths. Ottaviani writes

> In the cities where a great part of the citizens do not profess the Catholic Faith or do not even know the fact of Revelation, the non-Catholic civil authority must, in matters of religion, conform at least to the precepts of the natural law. Under these conditions, this non-Catholic authority should concede civil liberty to all the forms of worship that are not opposed to natural religion.[5]

"Natural religion" includes the truths and practices that man knows by reason with regard to God, including His existence, goodness, and providence; to reality, that it was created and is sustained

---

"'Constitution on the Church': A Schema Proposed by the Theological Commission; Second Part, Chapter IX: On the Relations between the Church and the State and On Religious Tolerance," no. 3, https://www.tradsurvivalguide.com/resources/they-have-uncrowned-him/chapter-34/.

[5] Ibid., no. 7.

and ruled by God; and to man, that he has an immortal soul that will be judged by God after death. "Civil society must therefore honor and serve God," as Ottaviani writes. In a "pluralistic" society where people hold a variety of religious beliefs, even if the vast majority of them are godless in practice and implication due to the overarching established ideology of liberalism, the civil authority is still obliged to honor and serve the True God. It does this by conforming its laws and norms to the natural moral law, and promoting and establishing only those religious beliefs, practices, and authorities in conformity with the natural theology I described above. The other "religions" it has the duty to proscribe, even to the extent of making them illegal.

Now, though not the corporate acceptance of Baptism and the establishment of the Catholic Church as the supreme moral and spiritual authority over the state, the stance taken by the civil authorities described above is certainly not neutral to God and religious truth, as it is in secular liberalism; let alone is it idolatry. And thus, it is pleasing to God. The demons would be held at bay by the presence of and recognition of true spiritual authority by the civil authority, albeit without complete understanding and rectitude, through the political order being ordered to God and as much moral and spiritual truth as is possible under the circumstances. It would be the same, morally speaking, as a non-Catholic individual doing his best to form and obey his conscience, though for the time being bereft of the true Faith due to no deliberate fault of his own. Such would be pleasing in God's sight, and hopefully, he would eventually discover and love the whole truth.

But Liberalism makes a mockery of all this by portraying its systematic and deliberate political godlessness and disobedience to the authority of the natural law as *good*, translated as inclusive, free and equal, tolerant, secular, and pluralistic. And this is true for all the variants of liberalism, both leftist social justice warriors and rightist libertarians. Both groups exclude the True (the truths of natural religion) and the Good (the natural moral law) from political authority, requiring the coercive power of the state to be employed only to secure "personal freedom" or "individual or collective rights," or "the general welfare," or the "will of the people," however these may be differently construed. But this is not pleasing to God, for it is a sin against reason, practical reason, whose first command is "Do good and avoid evil." The Good, not the Right, is the authority for all use of coercive power in the state, and the Good demands, as stated before, public recognition and obedience to God and the natural law. It does not require obedience to the mere will of men, even if it is the majority's will. The problem is not that we have an elite oligarchy imposing its will on the majority; the problem is that human will itself has been established and institutionalized as the ultimate authority, both individually and politically. It is this classical liberalism, now logically morphed into global totalitarianism—for both are grounded in nothing but the human will detached from any publicly recognized, transcendent moral and spiritual authority— that has invited the demons that now rule us through their human proxies.

We will never be able to exorcise these demons by attempting to replace them with "medical freedom," "individual sovereignty," or "the will of the people." These are counterfeit replacements for a freedom based upon the truth about human persons with immortal souls teleologically ordered to the natural and supernatural good, the sovereignty of the family, the Church, and all the natural communities that organically and corporately embody the common good and the will of God as known through the Logos, the Tao, the Natural Law. Now, I am a proponent of the natural, God-given freedoms and rights that legitimately authorize the use of political, coercive power to secure and protect them. But these freedoms and rights, properly understood as being grounded in natural and supernatural reality and interpreted definitively and authoritatively only by the Catholic Church, are not the same as the "American freedoms" granted to us, ostensibly, by the Declaration of Independence and the U.S. Constitution.

Though rhetorically our rights come from "Nature and Nature's God," there is no actual, historical religious tradition or institution to give determinate meaning and theological authority to such a claim, only unreal, ahistorical, abstract counterfeit of the actual tradition of the Catholic Church. As D.C. Schindler has demonstrated,[6] the "god" of the Declaration is not the Christian one, but an Enlightenment, deist, rationalist (and I would add, Freemasonic) substitute for the actual God of Abraham, Isaac, and Jacob, and of Jesus Christ. Thus, it has only as much authority as it has rhetorical and political power. It was quite easy for later generations of rulers to completely ignore and even reject this artificial civil theology when it was no longer persuasive, and to replace it with progressivism, secularism, and now Wokeism. Because there was no universally recognized transcendent moral and spiritual authority in the American Founding other than the Constitution and "We the People" (which meant,

---

[6] D.C. Schindler, *Freedom from Reality: The Diabolical Character of Modern Liberty* (Notre Dame, IN: University of Notre Dame Press, 2017).

in practice, the will of those empowered to represent the people—when we actually still had representative government—and now the will of psychopathic and Luciferian elites at war with the entire human race), American power, both domestically and abroad, is authorized by nothing but itself.

Thus, this power is uncheckable by anything other than an equal opposing power. But there is no such power at this time, and even if there were, it would inevitably employ its power under the conditions of modernity, meaning in a godless and self-referential manner. This is the main problem with the Catholic integralism of the Adrian Vermeule and Gladden Pappin variety—it is essentially Catholic Hobbesianism, with the true spiritual authority of the Church desacralized and profaned by being used as an instrument for the will to power of those who would control the now hegemonic Catholic discourse and thus decide what Catholicism means legally and politically.

It's not that we have been gradually losing our rights, freedoms, and political power since, say, the Civil War, and have now lost just about all of them under the plandemic totalitarianism. It's that we never really had them to begin with, for they were never grounded in true political authority. For true political authority is and must be grounded in reality, which in turn is nothing but a participation in transcendent spiritual reality and authority—and love—of God. The ultimate authority of God was revealed to us in its most pure form when it was utterly powerless, Jesus Christ Crucified. As the Church enters into her Passion in imitation of her Savior, we must be prepared to stay and suffer with her as she is crucified by the Powers and Principalities of the world under Antichrist, having been given up to them and him by the Antichurch Judases, who will be revealed as such. We must be able to recognize and submit to true authority precisely when it is utterly powerless, as Mary and John did, and to unmask and reject counterfeit authority when it is, seemingly, all-powerful. Begin by practicing it—now.

Well-being vs Salvation

Behind a burning red fog
The great mind swims in confusion
Its blood ferments in anger
Honor and wisdom will cower
Your river's flow is damned all to hell
Your river's flow is damned all to hell
Drifting in a current to stagnate
Encircle the vision of rust
Your river's flow is damned all to hell
Your river's flow is damned all to hell
Strong hearts soar through blindness
Tearing the fog, tearing the eyes
To clarity
To a place where truth is seen
Your shell is hollow, your shell is hollow, so am I
The rest will follow, the rest will follow, so will I
So will I. [7]

---

[7] Neurosis, "Under the Surface," on *Through Silver in Blood*, Neurot Recordings, 1996.

In his book entitled, *Marriage: Dead or Alive*, the twentieth-century, Swiss, Jungian psychiatrist, Adolf Guggenbühl-Craig, explained that marriage was failing more than ever before because it was mistakenly portrayed, understood, and practiced in the mode of *well-being*, where in truth it is a relationship and institution grounded in and ordered to *salvation*:

> Clearly not belonging to the state of well-being are tensions, dissatisfactions, painful emotions, anxiety, hatred, difficult and insoluble internal and external conflicts, obsessive searching for an undiscoverable truth, confused struggles about God, and the felt need to come to terms with evil and death. Sickness most certainly does not belong to the state of well-being. It is much easier, at any rate, for physically and psychologically healthy people to enjoy a sense of well-being than it is for the sick. "Give us our daily bread" really implies, "Give us daily our sense of well-being.". . . As goals, salvation and well-being contradict each other. The path to happiness does not necessarily include suffering. For the sake of our well-being, we are urged to be happy and not to break our heads with questions that have no answer. A happy person sits at the family table among loved ones and enjoys a hearty meal. A person who seeks salvation wrestles with God, the Devil, and the world, and confronts death, even if all of this is not absolutely necessary at that precise moment.[8]

---

[8] Adolf Guggenbühl-Craig, *Marriage: Dead or Alive*, rev. ed. (Woodstock, CT: Spring Publications, 2001), 25-26.

The mode of salvation was modeled perfectly for us in the life of Jesus Christ, and it is only by following His model that we can attain our soul's salvation. However, this is not to say that the salvation mode of life only became known to us by the Incarnation. It was known to the ancient Jews as well as the pagans, and it is known to today's Jews, Muslims, pagans, and secular humanists, for it is a fundamental part of natural human consciousness. Those who prefer this mode over the mode of well-being, and live it unto the end, are saved, regardless of what they know or do not know about Jesus Christ, unless, of course, they reject Him knowingly and deliberately. But if they are truly living within the mode of salvation, they will never do that. When Jesus comes to them three times before they die, as He told St. Faustina He would, they will recognize Him as the unknown Someone they had always been looking for, and the reason they ultimately rejected the mode of well-being for the much less comfortable mode of salvation.

A good pagan example of the two modes in contrast is found in the two heroes of Homer's epics, Achilles and Odysseus. Achilles is given a choice to live a long life of well-being or a short life of salvation. The mode of salvation for the warrior was a life of valor on the battlefield, seeking honor and glory more than the mere preservation of one's life. Achilles fulfilled this mode excellently until he was deprived of the honor he deserved by King Agamemnon. Achilles reacted with a superhuman rage and offense at this affront, and this not mainly because his war-trophy bride, Briseis, was taken from him, but more because he was destined before birth to have been the new Zeus, but was deprived of this by Zeus himself. According to a Pindaric tradition, Thetis, at the behest of Zeus, acceded to marriage with the mortal Peleus instead of Zeus in order to avert the birth of a son who would be stronger than his father. Achilles would have surpassed Zeus if his mother had not consented to a marriage beneath her divine status that neutralized the threat he constituted to Zeus's order. Achilles knew this, and so harbored in the recesses of his soul an infinite desire for divine power and glory that could never be satisfied, as well as an infinite divine rage at this existential frustration. This is an excellent image of the desire all humans have for divinization, along with the nagging sense that we were all destined for greatness but somehow lost it, and the ineradicable feeling of futility, dissatisfaction, and guilt with a mere life of well-being. Until Jesus came, we had no real ground for hope that our infinite longings could ever be fulfilled, yet some before Christ, such as faithful Hebrews and noble pagans, still chose to live as best they could in the mode of salvation, mysteriously knowing they were obliged to do so even without a grounded hope in an eventual successful end. Getting back to Achilles, when he was dishonored by Agamemnon, a mere mortal, it was as if his whole *raison d'etre* was destroyed, and he chose to leave the battle and live the mode of well-being in his tent, hanging out with his friends and playing music. To the Greek leaders who come to his tent to try to convince him to rejoin the battle, Achilles says:

> Neither Agamemnon nor any other Greek will change my mind, for it seems there is no gratitude for ceaseless battle with our enemies. He who fights his best and he who stays away earn the same reward, the coward and the brave man win like honor, death comes alike to the idler and to

him who toils. No profit to me from my sufferings, end-
lessly risking my life in war.[9]

Here Achilles reveals the mode of well-being he has recently
adopted, with its irrefutable logic of the futility of a life pursuing salvation (which, for the Mycenean Greek meant a short life of warrior
virtue). For those living at the time of the Trojan War, 1200 BC or
so, the afterlife in the underworld was a shadowy thing, neither punishment nor reward but a flittering, ghostlike, and passionless existence, barely alive, with no drama or purpose. In the *Odyssey*, Odysseus meets Achilles in the underworld and is told by him that so
lame is it down here that it is better to be a slave on the earth than to
rule Hades, in other words, that there is no reason to pursue the life
of salvation. But somehow, in spite of the nihilistic yet airtight, well-
being logic he entertains—what good is it to be a warrior if in death
all are equal, and equally half-dead?—Achilles knows that a life of
honor and courage and death-defying valor is ineluctably obligatory
for him, and that it violates a primordial, cosmic law for him to allow
his fellow Greeks to die dishonorably. And so when his best friend
Patroclus dies in battle due to his wallowing in well-being despair,
he re-establishes himself in salvation mode and kicks much Trojan
ass bedecked with god-designed armor and a shield that contains the
whole cosmos, signifying that the way of salvation, and not the way
of well-being, is written into the very fabric of things. And he dies
soon after by an arrow in his heel, as the later legends tell us.

---

[9] Homer, *The Iliad*, trans. Richmond Lattimore (Chicago: University of Chicago Press, 1951), Book 9, lines 378–379

Odysseus lived a salvation mode until, on his way home from Troy, he is waylaid by a nymph goddess, Calypso, who "traps" him on her island for seven years. I put *trap* in scare quotes because in the less-literal yet, I think, more accurate reading, Odysseus was free to leave anytime he wanted, and it is just the case that he did not want to, as he now had a matchless goddess as a very willing wife, and one who shared her immortality with him to boot. But her name means "she who conceals," and the price he had to pay for his well-being on steroids was never again to be seen and known by others, now or in the future, to have his life up till then never sung by bards to the future generations of Greeks. Somehow, he knew (when he got the seven-year itch) that risking abominable suffering and death in unknown waters populated by horrendous monsters with a very uncertain prospect of ever getting home alive was worth more than an eternity of perfect, earthly well-being. So, he built a raft and eventually got home, but not before singing his own song on the island of the Phaeacians, a paradisal mecca of well-being, whose king, Calypso-like, invited him to renounce his salvation, marry his beautiful daughter, and stay forever with them before sailing him (almost) home on a magic ship.

My last example from the ancient world is Job. According to the theology of his day, which was most probably after the Flood but well before Moses, those who followed God's law were blessed with a life of well-being, and this was a reason as good as any other to do so. If one did not experience well-being—health, long life, wealth, and a big family with lots of land and flocks—it meant that one was not pleasing to God, and deserved not to have it. But this was a mistaken notion of the economy of God and the true purpose for following Him, as Job was to discover. Satan challenged God by saying, essentially: "The only reason anyone 'loves' you and doesn't curse you is because you reward them with well-being. Take away their well-being and see what happens. You talk about salvation all the time. Well, they never really choose it, if it even exists. There is only well-being disguised as salvation." God aims to prove Satan wrong by taking away all the well-being from Job, and his counselors, of course, tell him it's because he has displeased God and urge him to repent of his sin. They are firmly in the well-being mode. Perhaps Job was as well at some time or another, but now he meditated for a long time on the dung heap, and he emerged in salvation mode, as he cried, "I know my redeemer lives." How did he know that? Everyone in the salvation mode knows it, and it is knowing it that puts one into salvation mode. He eventually was given his well-being back, but an intimate meeting with the unknowable God was what he wanted all along, and he got it: a terrifying whirlwind cross-examination that almost killed him. He didn't get a comprehensible and satisfying answer to the mystery of suffering, as the mode of well-being would expect. What he got was confirmation that salvation is not at all about human well-being or the lack of it, or even being just or unjust, pious or impious. It's something way beyond mere morality, however essential that is. It's about God, period. As St. Louis de Montfort often said: "God alone."

Why not just call these modes religious or non-religious, or even Christian or non-Christian? It is because those who practice religion and identify as such are not necessarily living the mode of salvation, and those who say they are not religious are not necessarily living the mode of well-being. People can say they believe in God and engage in external worship and seem to live for Him while living completely or mainly in the mode of well-being, and people can say that they don't believe or care about God or spiritual matters, and appear to everyone else not to, while living completely or mainly in the salvation mode. It seems to me that the well-being/salvation modes are more fundamental and definitive than the religious/non-religious labels, or even the self-identification of Christian or non-Christian. For, they are existential and primary, residing and operating in the deepest recesses of the heart and the will, invisible to all but God. Before we consciously choose to act at any specific time in any particular way, we have always already chosen, as it were, one of these modes, and our choices from then on are derivative from and caused by that primordial choice. Why we choose one mode or the other and persist in it is ultimately a mystery.

If the reader is still wondering what exactly the modes of well-being and salvation are, that's ok, for I am as well. It's not possible to nail them down in precise language. They are too big and deep for language. The particular mode of thought, cast of concepts, and exigency of language we happen now to understand and employ derives from and is constituted by one of these modes or the other. There is no third. If we are in the mode of well-being, we see the world that way, and we will not only not understand the mode of salvation, we will despise it. Furthermore, we will not even recognize that we are in a mode at all—it is just the way things are. One has to be in the mode of salvation to understand that experiential modes even exist, and then to understand the nature of each mode and their radical opposition. For, these two modes determine exhaustively the very contours of the meaning of life itself, as they are the earthly images of the two modes of eternity. Thus, it must not be expected that they can be discretely and definitively defined in this life. They can be described, pointed to, adumbrated, suggested, intuited, exemplified, metaphorized, allegorized, unveiled, demarcated, translated, and cartographed—but never exhaustively grasped. It is these modes, after all, that define us.

The mode of well-being is a living hell that leads to eternal hell. The mode of salvation is a living heaven that leads to eternal heaven. And here is the most compelling reason I can think of why this is the case: Hell is the choice for the complete absence of God, Who is ultimate reality. Hell is thus the choice for ultimate unreality. Thus, the mode of well-being chosen in this life is a life of perpetual and absolute war with ultimate reality. We live within a global culture of well-being, an elite-imposed and artificial, totalitarian therapeutic prison, and this means that through an ineluctable cultural conditioning process, well-being is the default position of the collective consciousness. Charles Taylor calls it the Immanent Frame, and we are meant by our puppeteer conditioners to know of nothing other, just as they know nothing other. If we do not deliberately fight to resist and escape this conditioning, it will mold and poison our souls unconsciously. But even if we somehow become acquainted while within this prison with the salvific mode of consciousness, through, say, encountering traditional religion or reading classic literature or meeting a living saint, we are programmed to translate this experience into the discourse, grammar, and social-imaginary of well-being, thereby turning it into its opposite.

And this includes everyone, whether traditional Catholic, fundamentalist Christian, Koranic mystic, alt-right groyper, paleocon-bearded hipster, dark web gnostic, or perennialist blackpiller, all of which would seem quite immune to such conditioning and who would certainly, it seems, reject the default position. The mode of well-being has been firmly in place in the West for centuries, and it has been getting ever more well-being-ish ever since, exponentially since the year 2020. Medieval Christendom was a culture of salvation. Well-being as a plausible mode of life didn't exist, and if one chose it, one knew he was choosing hell. This is what wicked people do. People sinned, of course, by choosing well-being against salvation, but they were ashamed of it, and society let them know. Modernity, on the other hand, is a culture of well-being as the Good, a culture in which the mode of salvation is utterly shameful—fanatical, intolerant, superstitious, fundamentalist, antisemitic.

Perhaps an example of this will be helpful. The plandemic of 2020 was a test, a trial run for the Final Judgment deciding the eternity of every human being ever to live, either Heaven or Hell. What was placed before every human being at the time was a stark existential and theological choice, a choice that was also a judgment. For those for whom this trial would be the manifestation and confirmation of their prior existential choice for well-being or the uberchoice of their preferred long-term state, it seemed no choice at all. I mean, there was a deadly virus, you know, the deadliest one, and all you needed to do to avoid your own sickness or death and prevent the sickness and death of others was to do what you were told to do by those authorized to protect you from sickness and death. If you did that, the curve would be flattened. They told you to allow certain others to stick a swab in your nose, wear a mask all day, stay six feet away from other people, stay home, and close your business or school or church. They were so loving and committed to your health that they painfully coerced these directives, rewarding you if you obeyed them and punishing you if you did not. They told you to get the vaccine or else you would most probably die and kill others, and they helped you to make the right choice by making sure that your life would be a living hell if you refused the shot.

The problem is that if you chose to do what they told you, you were not choosing to protect yourself and others from a deadly virus. What you really were choosing is hell. Now, there were some who were genuinely invincibly ignorant to the lies they were believing, at least at first, and so not culpable. But in the weeks and months after, as reality reasserted itself, it became impossible to believe the lies without fault. You were choosing hell because you were choosing unreality, and knowingly so. By choosing to obey arbitrary and irrational prescriptions you were choosing to believe in the Big Lie that underlay them, namely, that healthy people with no symptoms of illness are contagious. You, of course, knew this to be untrue. Everyone knows this to be untrue. But you believed it anyway and acted accordingly. And you were quite proud of your mendacious insanity. You believed this insane lie because it made you feel good, in both the pleasurable and moral meaning of the word, but in doing so you put yourself under false authority. And you knew that it was false authority. No one thinks that healthy people with no symptoms are contagious, not even you. But you thought it anyway. "Just wear the f$%*in mask"—the first commandment of Hell. You obeyed this commandment with diabolical pleasure and took the same pleasure in torturing and scapegoating those who disobeyed it. Now, not everyone behaved this maliciously, and I am describing the extreme covidiot here, but all of us to some extent participated in this treasonous, hell-worthy behavior.

Is putting oneself under false authority really so bad? Yes, it is the worst sin possible. It is the sin against the Holy Spirit, which Jesus said is unforgivable. It is calling good evil and evil good. Salvation comes from putting oneself under the authority of Truth, Who is Jesus Christ, the Son of the Father, Who was with God in the beginning and is God. Damnation comes from putting yourself under the authority of untruth, whose father is Satan, the father of lies, who was a liar and murderer from the beginning. And it is one's attitude to truth that distinguishes the mode of well-being from the mode of salvation. In well-being, one puts truth second to everything else. Truth is never first. Perhaps it is an authority, but it is never *the* authority. In salvation, truth is always first. It is Authority, period. One can seek well-being, for we are morally permitted to do so and our souls desire happiness, but it is always a striving for well-being and happiness in the light of and under the authority of truth. And if believing in and obeying the truth means that one's earthly well-being and happiness are sacrificed, then so be it. Salvation comes first. Salvation means eternal well-being, which is ultimately in tension with earthly well-being and happiness, but is all that matters in the end. Earthly well-being is a good, and those who live in the mode of salvation obtain it in its essence, which is joy and peace in union with God in this life, which no one can take away. Sometimes this joy and peace are accompanied by worldly goods, such as financial prosperity and bodily health and good reputation. But sometimes not. It doesn't matter one way or the other for the salvation-minded. Obedience to truth is all that matters. For the well-being-minded, a feeling of well-being is all that matters, and knowing and obeying truth is, at best, only a means to this highest end.

The Catholic Church is the mode of salvation on Earth, for it is the mystical body of the Incarnate Savior. If this mode existed in cultures before Christ and His Church, it was solely due to His providential grace in anticipation of and preparation for His Church, the soul and lifeblood of the world. At the present moment, the human infrastructure and clerical personnel of the Church, in league with her unbaptized external enemies, are at war with her divine core, and Satan is in control of the majority of the clerical human personnel and all of her external enemies. Satan's hegemony over the Church and thus the world has been building since the 1900s but really in earnest after 1962. Leo XIII and Our Ladies of Akita and Fatima had prophesized it and told us what to do to prevent it, but most didn't listen. What this means is that there has never been a time in the history of the human race in which the mode of salvation has been more eclipsed and difficult to live out, and the mode of well-being more pronounced, seductive, irresistible, ubiquitous, and easy to practice, than today. One might think of the time before Christ as comparable or even worse than now, but consider that the corruption of the best is the worst, that nothing could be worse than a counterfeit of salvation replacing the true one, and such could only be possible after the historical manifestation of the full salvific truth of Jesus Christ. What we have today is much worse than paganism, and much worse than even the most corrupt and "dark" of post-incarnation ages of years past. What we have is a culture of well-being that wears the mask of salvation, with the salvation mode counterfeited out of existence. Even the best of the salvation-mode sub-cultures of today are more or less compromised and tainted by the ubiquitous well-being culture, and they easily end up becoming mirror images of it, appearing to be solidly salvific but surreptitiously and subtly counterfeit. They talk salvation but walk well-being.

> This is all I've known
> A way to be
> True to all
> All that inspires
> A torch in a black sea
> Our stones still stand
> To remind us of loss
> A loss mirrored on our souls
> A watchfire brings strength
> Breathe in the heat
> In the eternal path
> Armored against life[10]

Human beings were created by God for happiness in the worship of God. For reasons entirely inscrutable to human beings, God decided to make this happiness a personal choice for which we are responsible. This means that humans can choose not to worship God, that is, choose unhappiness over happiness. Why would a human being choose unhappiness and reject the very reason he was created? No one knows the answer to this question, for it is a mystery, the

---

[10] Neurosis, "Watchfire," *Through Silver in Blood*, Relapse Records, 1996,

unfathomable and inscrutable mystery of evil. All we know is that we cannot escape this choice. Whether we obtain eternal happiness in the worship of God or eternal unhappiness in the refusal of this worship is entirely up to us, and any of us is capable of choosing against his own happiness. If you end up in hell for all eternity, it is because you wanted while alive and want now to be there. You refused to worship God, and you did so knowing it would mean eternal hell, and you chose it anyway.

What does the choice for hell look like? The Catholic Church teaches us that if we die in a state of unrepentance, in a state of mortal sin, we go to hell. What is it to commit a mortal sin, and what does a state of unrepentance look like? Jesus said, "You shall know the truth, and the truth shall set you free," and "I am the way, the truth, and the life. No one comes to the Father except through me." At its core, mortal sin is the refusal to know and obey truth, which is to say, to reject reality, for truth is the conformity of our souls with reality. At the core of reality is the Good, which is reality qua desirable. And since Jesus Christ is the truth, reality incarnate, then every refusal of reality, refusal to know and obey truth, is a rejection of Jesus, the Incarnate Good. Unrepentance means that we persist up to the moment of death in this rejection in the knowledge that we are choosing hell because of it. We end in up hell if we persist until the last in our rejection of reality, truth, and Jesus Christ.

Why would anyone reject reality and truth and the Good and Jesus Christ? For whatever reason, we are not in a right relationship with reality and so misunderstand the truth about it. We reject what we do not know is truth. This is certainly possible, but why do we

not know the truth? We are personally responsible for the relationship we have with reality in this life and when we die, and if it is not
the right one, it is ultimately our fault. Not knowing something is
the truth at one time or another can certainly be the fault of someone
else whom we depend on for knowing what is true, such as a parent
or a teacher or a culture, but this is a temporary and remediable situation. The injustice done to our souls by false authorities may not
be our fault, but we have the ability and responsibility to rectify this
injustice. Even though it is the case that reality is mediated to us by
human authorities that could be mistaken or lying about the truth,
and mediated by our own faculties of knowing that might be, due to
ourselves or others, damaged or faulty, this does not excuse us from
the personal responsibility of doing all we can to ensure that we are
in a correct relationship with reality and thus know what is true. And
we have the responsibility of not only knowing what is true, but also
loving and obeying it. If we did not have this responsibility, hell
would not exist, for we would always have a legitimate excuse that
renders us not personally responsible for our not knowing and not
loving truth. There would be no real guilt. But hell does exist.

How do we overcome the damage done to our souls by others
and ourselves that has caused us, right now, not to be in a right relationship with reality and thus not to know or love what is true?
Since we are dependent on others for knowing certain truths, and
even for the development in us, especially when we are young, of the
habit of being docile to truth, how do we overcome this dependency
when it has led us into a soul-state of untruth? The answer is that we
are always able to choose between well-being, in which truth isn't a
priority, and salvation, where it is the only priority, regardless of

how badly we might have been damaged. Indeed, if we had always chosen salvation over well-being, we would not be damaged right now in the first place, for when in a state of salvation, we are immune to the damage done to our souls by the truth-treason of others. The problem is, of course, that we were not and are not now fully in a state of salvation, and so have been damaged. But we can begin to undo this damage by choosing, right now, to be in the salvation mode, and we can keep choosing until the moment we die.

Consider the situation of a Pharisee at the time of Christ. He was badly damaged by the Jewish culture in which he was raised, for it was thoroughly corrupt, even though it was given to the Jews by God Himself. Jesus gives a very clear picture of this culture:

But woe to you, scribes and Pharisees, hypocrites! For you lock people out of the kingdom of heaven. For you do not go in yourselves, and when others are going in, you stop them. Woe to you, scribes and Pharisees, hypocrites! For you cross sea and land to make a single convert, and you make the new convert twice as much a child of hell as yourselves. Woe to you, scribes and Pharisees, hypocrites! For you clean the outside of the cup and of the plate, but inside they are full of greed and self-indulgence. You blind Pharisee! First clean the inside of the cup, so that the outside also may become clean. . . . Woe to you, scribes and Pharisees, hypocrites! For you are like whitewashed tombs, which on the outside look beautiful, but inside they are full of the bones of the dead and of all kinds of filth. So you also on the outside look righteous

to others, but inside you are full of hypocrisy and lawlessness.[11]

Imagine being raised as a Pharisee in this culture. It was a culture
of well-being, not salvation, due to the Jewish leaders' treason
against God. No Pharisee was forced to participate in this corrupt
culture, for he still had access to uncorrupted scriptures and traditions. He could have resisted the corruption and even called it out,
as Jesus did, but this would have required consistently being in and
acting from the mode of salvation, which would have been quite difficult with all the pressure to and rewards from being in the mode of
well-being masking as the mode of salvation. Who was modeling it
for them? No one. It was the opposite. The Pharisee leaders were
modeling Satan, whom Jesus called their father. But Jesus, the perfect embodiment of the uncorrupted scriptures and tradition, was
now present in their midst; now they had a model and thus the ability to compare themselves to the Good and see and repent of their
evil. He made their evil quite clear to them, and there was no reason
not to believe Him, for He had no hypocrisy in Him, and He spoke
to them in love and from the mode of salvation. Perhaps before Jesus
came they had some excuse for their evil, but not now. All a Pharisee
had to do was to pose one question to himself: "Is He the evil one,
or is it I?" This is a question anyone at any time can ask, and it is a
question evoked by the existential mode of salvation, a mode anyone
at any time can adopt in the deepest recesses of his soul.

Saul became Paul when he adopted this mode and asked this
question, a question prompted by a shocking mystical encounter

---

[11] Matthew 23:13–15, 25–28 (NRSV)

with the Risen Lord that knocked him to the ground and left him physically blind. God will always provide the precise experiences we need to get into the salvation mode and begin asking salvific questions, but only if we first desire to exist in the mode by which such questions will be salvific. Saul must have desired this in the core of his being, and Jesus saw this and helped him to fulfill it. Jesus knew how evil the culture was that produced Saul the Christ-hating Pharisee, and He provided him a way out. Of course, the desire and ability to live in the salvific mode is itself a gift of God unmerited by us without which we could never be saved. But it is always offered and made available to us. We must simply choose it.

A good culture is one that forms its denizens to be in a right relationship to reality, causing the mind to know it and the will to love it. A good culture makes it easier to know and love truth, and a bad culture makes it harder. The Pharisee culture of the Jews in Saul's day was a bad culture, for it disposed its leaders to reject Jesus Christ. The rejection of Jesus Christ is at the very heart of Western culture in our day and has been so for a long time, though harder to recognize in past centuries. Our present culture makes it very easy not to know and love truth, for it makes it all but impossible and undesirable to ask questions from the mode of salvation, especially this question: "Is it true?" It thus makes it very easy to be, live, and act in the mode of well-being while thinking one is in the mode of salvation, or not even knowing that there is any other mode than well-being, or that one is in any "mode" at all. How can we be saved from this most perilous deception? Alasdair MacIntyre:

We have within our social order few if any social milieus within which reflective and critical enquiry concerning the central issues of human life can be sustained.... This tends to be a culture of answers, not of questions, and those answers, whether secular or religious, liberal or conservative, are generally delivered as though meant to put an end to questioning.[12]

Paul Evdokimov:

The outdated religious person and the modern sophisticated irreligious individual meet back to back in an immanence imprisoned within itself.... The denial of God has thus permitted the affirmation of man. Once this affirmation is effected, there is no longer anything to be denied or subordinated... On this level total man will not be able to ask any questions concerning his own reality, just as God does not put a question to himself.[13]

There are only two paths in life, the one that leads to heaven and the one that leads to hell. And there are only two modes of living, salvation and well-being. One must live in the mode of salvation to end up in heaven, and living exclusively the mode of well-being can

---

[12] Alasdair MacIntyre, *The Tasks of Philosophy: Volume 1: Selected Essays* (Cambridge: Cambridge University Press, 2006), 182.

[13] Paul Evdokimov, *The Struggle with God*, trans. Sister Gertrude, S.P. (Glen Rock, NJ: Paulist Press, 1966), 5.

only lead to hell. Heaven begins on earth when one pursues salvation, and hell is also here for those who only pursue well-being. One cannot live in both modes, as they are mutually exclusive, though one can live in one and then another. It is the mode that one persists in until the end that determines eternity. It is not that well-being is hell per se, for it is a good, though not the ultimate one, and the fruit of living the mode of salvation is true well-being in this life, the most that is possible on earth, a life of sometimes agonizing and unspeakable suffering, surely, but also ineffable peace, supernal joy, and indomitable hope. Living in God's Divine Will is heaven itself, and it begins now. And it culminates in eternity with the most well-being possible to a creature, complete union with God. So, well-being is good, but if we seek it and not God as our main goal in this life, if it is our primary existential mode, with salvation taking a back seat, we obtain neither well-being nor salvation.

The totalitarians ruling us are Satanists, whether officially or not, and they want to abuse us to such an extent that we no longer ask questions in the mode of salvation in obedience to the ultimate authority of Truth and thereby save our souls. Asking questions indicates a soul that is aware of her dignity as a responsible creature, personally responsible to know and obey the authority of truth, not human counterfeits of it. The Satanists want us to degrade ourselves by choosing idols over God, and they want us to do so knowingly and deliberately. This is why they hate questions more than anything. Ultimately, they want us to feel we are so worthless and stupid and deserving of nothing but abuse and death that we voluntarily murder ourselves. They'd rather we do it to ourselves, for it would mean more souls in hell. The first step to obtaining their goal is to get us to stop asking questions and caring about the Truth. God is the answer to all questions. They want us to see them as God. If we stop asking questions about the claims and actions of any human being, we are obeying their satanic command. Origen once wrote: "Every true question is like the lance which pierces the side of Christ causing blood and water to flow forth."[14] It is the blood and water that saved the Centurion, and it will save us if we so desire it. All we need to do is continually ask ourselves these questions: "Is it true? Am I pursuing salvation right now, or well-being?" And God will do the rest.

State Sorcery, Pathocracy, and the Traitors among Us

When an explanation for a massively violent event and its concomitant crisis emerges as the official, unquestionable, and authoritative narrative; when it includes, and without empirical evidence or investigative inquiry, the assignation of innocence and exceptionalism of the victims, and utter depravity and terrifying power to the designated criminals; when dissent from this narrative is socially forbidden, even to the extent of legal harassment and prosecution; when it spawns behavior in contradiction with itself, such as committing acts of terror in the name of eradicating terrorism,

---

[14] Quoted in Archbishop Bruno Forte, "Religion and Freedom: Searching For the Infinitely Loving Father-Mother," a lecture given at a meeting of the bishops of England and Wales, Nov. 12, 2007, available at: http://www.catholic.org/featured/headline.php?ID=5262.

or restricting and punishing free speech in the name of expanding and protecting it; when the narrative is immediately supported, echoed, and policed by the vast majority of the ruling classes, including both the mainstream and 'alternative' (gate-keeping left and right; when it successfully unites and synthesizes otherwise opposed factions of the populace—liberals with neoconservatives, libertarians with statists, humanists with Nietzscheans, theists with atheists; when rational scrutiny and frank discussion of obvious explanation holes in the narrative are forbidden; and when the ritualistic, annual remembrance of an event and recitation of its hallowed story—particularly the harrowing portrayal of the demonic villains to which it assigns all blame for both the increasing domestic strife among citizens and the perpetual Manichean war against the newest 'enemy'—instils and evokes primordial fear and religious awe in the populace; when the narrative of an event or series of connected events possesses all of these attributes, or even just a few of them, we know we are dealing with no ordinary phenomenon.[15]

We stand encircled by wing and fire
Our deepest ties return and turn upon us
The shrouded reason, the bleeding answer
The human plague in womb
Bring clouds of war
Let us rest

---

[15] Thaddeus J. Kozinski, *Modernity as Apocalypse: Sacred Nihilism and the Counterfeits of Logos* (Brooklyn, NY: Angelico Press, 2019), 189-90.

Our future breed is the last
In the conscience waits
Dreams of the new sun
We're blood in the dust
Given to the Rising
Through this we claw roots
Of trees in the world of iron
Our father's steps fueled the boiling sea
The wretched harvest reaped by the hands of dawning
Our pain cannot forgive the silent machine of the fatal flaw
in man
That brings us to the end.[16]

We are in the end times. The Antichrist is coming, and many, perhaps most, will worship him unto destruction and damnation. The totalitarianism and wickedness will become unimaginable, resembling something worse than a synthesis of Hunger Games, Blade Runner, 1984, Brave New World, Mad Max, The Road, and The Matrix. The Catholic Church, as well as authentic Christians and men of earnest goodwill, will be starkly divided between a small remnant faithful to the Tao and Jesus Christ, the Mystical Body of Christ, and the large masses of Antichrist worshippers, the Mystical Body of the Devil, both within and without the institutional Church, which will attempt both to counterfeit and destroy the Remnant. The hell on earth that was the plandemic was just the prelude to this final apocalypse. Undoubtedly, the last four years were a severe and revelatory,

---

[16] Neurosis, "Given to the Rising," on *Given to the Rising*, released June 5, 2007, CD, Neurot Recordings.

global spiritual trial, with most Christians committing treason against their Lord and neighbor by scapegoating the innocent, wearing the slave mask, and taking the bioweapon, thereby deserving and ushering in the next and final onslaught as chastisement, which will be in truth a last-ditch effort of God's love and mercy, but will be experienced by most as inexorable and unforgiving wrath.

If what I am saying is true, what shall we do to prepare ourselves? Physically and economically, we need to do what we can to become as self-sustaining as possible and to live on the margins, lest we be complicit with and coopted by a Techno-Leviathan-Antichrist-System that will be ubiquitous and inescapable. There will be no place to run, really, but we need to get out of the main Sodoms. But the most important reason to prepare is not for the sake of temporal and material well-being, though this is essential, but to safeguard our psychological sanity and spiritual integrity. Just as it was in the plandemic, the target of the evil was not primarily our bodies but our souls, and his main strategy was to get us, through fear, fraud, or seduction, to commit the unforgivable sin. "Woe to you that call evil good, and good evil: that put darkness for light, and light for darkness: that put bitter for sweet, and sweet for bitter" (Isaiah 5:20). This is the sin of idolatry, which is unforgivable precisely because it makes repentance impossible. When we are in the throes of idolatry, we see good as evil and evil as good, and we do so, to some extent at least, knowingly and deliberately. No one worships an idol unknowingly or accidentally. "I will not worship God, but I will worship this!" There can be no greater obstacle to salvation than idolatry, and this is why, as St. Thomas Aquinas tells us, when Jesus prayed, "Father, forgive them for they know not what they do," the Pharisees were not included. They knew Whom they crucified. They were idolaters of power, calling Goodness Itself evil.

And idolatry is never just a private, personal sin. It is always bound up with the social, cultural, and political, meaning that personal idolatry is always already public idolatry, and vice-versa. If a social and political order is not based upon God, it will be based upon an idol—there is no empty shrine. And, as Aristotle, taught, the "good citizen" of this regime will be the state idolater, whether the idol is honor, money, freedom, or power. The criminals will be identified as those who refuse to worship the idol, and treated accordingly. Liberalism, which insists that its coercive legal power is always "secular" and "neutral" regarding moral and spiritual truth, is a lie created in the depths of Hell. Either truth, especially supernatural truth, is publicly recognized, obeyed, and made the foundation of the laws and customs of a country, or lies, especially diabolical and blasphemous ones, will be established surreptitiously, coercively, and in a totalitarian manner.

What is the evidence for this? Philosophically and theologically, it's found in the *philosophia perennis* and the infallible social and political theology of the Catholic Church. Historically, it's found in the fact that all political orders *ab initio* have been religiously founded and exclusivist, including those whose political rhetoric served to hide this fact, the "secular liberal democracies" since the late 18th and early 19th centuries. And since Protestantism is intrinsically self-defeating and anarchic, with the ultimate religious authority enshrined in the individual believer, it entrenched an airtight practical logic whose complete unfolding, with the help of Freemasonry and other occult groups, would eventually mandate that only anti-Christian and anti-Tao forms of religion, such as the religion of liberalism itself, would have exclusive legal and political authority and thus the sole justification for coercive legal and political power.

But if you don't buy the philosophical, theological, and historical evidence, the empirical evidence over the past four years is overwhelming, self-evident, and irrefutable, at least to those who haven't yet been fully indoctrinated and soul-washed by the now thoroughly established official religion of . . . well, the best word for it is the religion of the Antichrist. It's liberalism, yes, but now without its mask of neutrality. Sodomy, usury, mass murder, genocide, child-mutilation and child sacrifice—these are not new sins, and all the ancient pagan regimes practiced them, but when were they ever endorsed in the name of Christian love and human dignity? A totalitarian hell on earth was created by Luciferian billionaires, and the mind-control, mass trauma, mass psychosis, mass murder, unprecedented economic destruction, suspension of established legal and customary rights, and global theft by elites of trillions from the middle class was and is still celebrated by many Americans, and most Catholic Bishops rationalized it all as responsible and caring policies following "the science" and for "safety"—with the occupier of the Chair of Peter having commanded all of us to inject ourselves with a deadly bioweapon as an act of love. And just when this onslaught subsided (the screws have been loosened temporarily, following the professional torturer's playbook), we add blasphemy and sacrilege to the litany of state-sponsored religious practices, with child-grooming (drag-queen story hour) publicly endorsed as "diversity education," homosexuals dressed as nuns simulating sodomy on a crucifix pub-

licly honored by a professional baseball team as "community heroes," and those who choose to use the anus as a sex organ are given
a feast day, nay, a feast month, in the satanic state's religious calen-
dar, replacing the month devoted to the Sacred Heart. And there is
the unspeakable Israeli genocide of Palestinians done right out in the
open and celebrated by millions of American "Christians."

And what is worst of all is the emergence of a group of traitorous
Catholic intelligentsia—they call themselves "progressives." Their
main job is to slander, mock, and character assassinate any Catholic
who publicly defends Catholic truth and morals and condemns the
spiritual atrocities that they defend with a smarmy and mendacious
Christian gloss. There are such diabolical groups in every organization that resist the satanic-state religion. Every God-fearing-and-
obeying institution or community had been infiltrated by these minions of the Devil. These Judas Catholics just can't wait to hand over
faithful Catholics to today's Herods and Pilates. It starts with scapegoating and demonizing fellow Catholics. When they have been
thoroughly demonized on Catholic social media according to the official enemy designations of the Regime—"homophobic," "white supremacist," "extremist," "racist," "conspiracy theorist," "anti-
semite,"—the sheep are then at the mercy of the wolves. The FBI and
the Department of Justice has systematically targeted and arrested
Catholic "terrorists" who happen simply to have been publicly pro-
life.[17] The Antichurch Judases are aligned with the ADL's evil agenda

[17] https://www.catholicnewsagency.com/news/253523/acquitted-pro-life-ac-
tivist-mark-houck-reveals-details-of-fbi-raid-will-press-charges.
https://www.ncregister.com/cna/mark-houck-and-wife-sue-fbi-and-doj-for-ma-
licious-prosecution-era-of-targeting-pro-lifers-is-over. E. Michael Jones, "How I
Landed on the FBI Hit List: Targeting Radical Traditionalist Catholics," *Culture*

by their own mendacious and spiteful targeting of faithful, pro-life Catholics on social media.

The assault on Reality comes mostly from above, from the elite puppeteers, constituted by psychopaths and Luciferians, and their motivation is pure malice and pure power. And they have created institutional structures, such as stakeholder global capitalism, "diversity, inclusion, and equity" czars, and hate-speech laws, that mirror the evil in their souls and thus serve to cultivate evil in the masses through their unwitting or witting participation in them. Both the elite cabal and these institutions rule us, and it's hard to see where one ends and the other begins. It is important to note that both the elites and the institutions wouldn't have any real power over the masses if they didn't employ moralistic propaganda to cloak their true intentions and the intentions of these institutions. Non-psychopaths and non-devil-worshippers cannot fathom the extent and depth of their personal malice and that of the institutions they and their useful idiots employ, for such evil is the thing of stories, they insist, living only in horror movies, a few psychotic serial killers, and mythical monsters.

In 1984 (interestingly enough), a Polish psychiatrist named Andrzej Łobaczewski (1921-2007) completed the work that he began shortly after World War II as a member of a group of social scientists studying the nature of totalitarianism, having experienced it firsthand first under Nazism and then Stalinism. The book that was the fruit of his many years of suffering and research is *Political Ponerology: A Science on the Nature of Evil Adjusted for Political Purposes.*[18]

Wars, March, 2023.

[18] Andrzej Łobaczewski, *Political Ponerology: The Science of Evil, Psychopathy,*

His thesis was that the regimes he suffered under, including to some extent the United States to which he immigrated in the late 1970s, are most accurately described as pathocracies, ruled by a small group of genetic psychopaths, with a wider group of willing lackeys with psychopathic tendencies, creating a political culture of "acquired psychopathy." The masses are duped by the Orwellian distortion of language—deadly bioweapons are "safe and effective, child mutilation is "gender affirming surgery"—that both enables and accompanies pathocratic rule, for normal people naturally characterize and translate any pathological behavior and speech into the moral and rational categories with which they are familiar due to their inability to imagine the psychological world in which the psychopaths live. As Łobaczewski's Polish colleague Stefan Błachowski wrote:

> The general inability to recognize the psychological type of such individuals [i.e. psychopaths] causes immense suffering, mass terror, violent oppression, genocide and the decay of civilization. … As long as the suggestive [i.e. hypnotic, charming, 'spellbinding'] power of the psychopaths is not confronted with facts and with moral and practical consequences of his doctrine, entire social groups may succumb to his demagogic appeal. . . .Methods are developed for spreading dissension between groups (as in the maxim 'divide et impera' [divide and rule]."[19]

and the Origins of Totalitarianism (Red Pill Press, 2022).

[19] Dąbrowski, K. (with Kawczak, A. & Sochanska, J.), The Dynamics of Concepts (London: Gryf, 1973), pp. 40, 47. Dąbrowski, K. 1996 [1977]. 'Multilevelness of Emotional and Instinctive Functions' (Lublin, Poland: Towarzystwo Naukowe Katolickiego Uniwersytetu Lubelskiego, 1996 [1977]), p. 33. Quoted in Harrison

Just as with the scamdemic, plain treason and malicious deceit in politics are given justification and are presented as positive values. Principles of taking advantage of concrete situations are also developed. Political murder, execution of opponents, concentration camps, and genocide are the product of political systems at the level of primary integration [i.e. psychopathy]. Needless to say, Łobaczewski was prophetic. IXXI, the genocidal War on Terror that it birthed, the scamdemic crimes against humanity, and the trans/pedo sexual assault on and corruption of children bear all the pathocratic earmarks described above. False-flag terrorism and deep-state psyops are intrinsically psychopathic, and yet they are now the normal modus operandi of contemporary politics. Due to the Internet and courageous truth-tellers, many are waking up to this fact.

But what we are dealing with in the twenty-first century is even worse than pathocracy. We are dealing with state sorcery. I believe the mass murder of millions and brainwashing of billions by the Covid psychological operation and bioweapon was also a mass ritual of sorcery. *Revelation* 18:23: "And the light of a candle shall shine no more at all in thee; and the voice of the bridegroom and of the bride shall be heard no more at all in thee: for thy merchants were the great men of the earth; for by thy sorceries were all nations deceived." The Greek word for "sorceries" in verse 23 is *"pharmakeia"* [far-mak-i'-ah]. According to the Thayer Greek Dictionary *"pharmakeia"* is "the use or administering of drugs; poisoning; and sorcery, magical arts, often found in connection with idolatry and fostered by it."[20]

Our pathocracy, and the Luciferianism that now accompanies and exacerbates it, can also be seen in the attempt of these elites to overthrow not only morality, in their promotion of homosexuality, trans-insanity, pedophilia, child-mutilation, and baby murder, but also Being itself, in their rejection of the immutable reality of gender and the intractable limits of human freedom. Yuval Harari, advisor to Klaus Schwab, tells us that "man is a hackable animal."[21] This is right out of chapter three of C.S. Lewis's *The Abolition of Man*, where an elite of "controllers" destroy all awareness of the Tao genetically, with future generations doomed to an imbecilic existence as slaves of the elites. In 2019, Ottawa's highest court legally prohibited a father from preventing his fourteen-year-old son from undergoing a sex-change operation.[22] This is a State at war with Being and anyone who dares to recognize the authority of Logos over the authority of the State. Both psychopaths and Satanists behave as if they are not creatures but gods and they are working to create a culture wherein their demented mode of consciousness becomes the mode of consciousness of all, with all those who resist either murdered or put into permanent concentration camps.

Metaphysically speaking, every human being is a person, an "I," not an "it," and morally speaking, we are obliged to treat both ourselves and others as "I's and not "its." Psychopaths and Luciferians

---

[20] Joseph Henry Thayer, *Thayer's Greek-English Lexicon of the New Testament*, 3rd ed. (Peabody, MA: Hendrickson Publishers, 1995).

[21] https://www.ynharari.com/commencement-speech-2020-congratulations-you-are-now-hackable-animals/.

[22] https://globalnews.ca/news/6399468/bc-gender-change-court/.

treat themselves as the only "I's" that exist, and everyone else as their "its." Liberalism is just the social, cultural, economic, political, and religious embodiment of the twisted soul of the psychopath and Luciferian, and when they are in power, they work tirelessly to habituate otherwise normal and moral people into the infernal consciousness and outlook of these demons in human form. This habituation is becoming global now. After IXXI, being a good person meant believing all government and mass-media narratives without any critical assessment, condoning the murder of Muslims and wars of genocidal aggression, and substituting secular ideologies for the Catholic Church as the only true "force for good in the world." During the plandemic, it meant obeying the science, staying home, turning in your neighbor for noncompliance, shutting down your business and your church, masking up yourself and your children, and getting the shot—in other words, submitting to physical and mental torture, bodily and spiritual enslavement. During the Ukraininsane, as I like to call it, it meant mindlessly hating Putin and supporting Ukraine—and the propaganda onslaught for this psy-op perhaps dwarfed even the plandemic propaganda, if that is possible, leading to the very real possibility of nuclear war, even now. In 2020, being a good American means bringing your children to be entertained by mentally and criminally insane pedophiles and paying "doctors" to chemically castrate them, if not physically cut off their penises and breasts. And now being a good American means supporting Israel, even when it commits deliberate genocide.

Why is God allowing what seems a full-scale demonic possession of the institutions and public space, along with many of the rulers, of our culture? The plandemic was pure diabolical mass-torture, and although many invited this torture, justified it, called it good—the sin against the Holy Spirit—and even celebrated it, going further and further into the hell their sins conjured, many woke up to the reality of Satan through it, for there could be no earthly explanation for the extent, depth, coordination and utter malice of the evil to which we were subjected. An exorcist of the Catholic Church, Fr. Chad Ripperger, has explained why God allows demons to oppress and possess people. The true reality of sin is an unimaginable horror, but God in His mercy would like us to avoid and detest sin for the sake of love of Him and neighbor. When we refuse to do this and become adjusted to a particular sin and evil behavior so that it becomes attractive, desirable, and even second nature to us, God must force us, as it were, to repent of it by making our life as miserable as possible; he allows a demon to torture us. The suffering is horrific, but we now hate the demon who tortures us, and we now know it's due to our sin, so we repent—hopefully. This repentance, with the help of the exorcist, allows the demon to be expelled. I wonder if the Western world is undergoing this "demonic therapy" to some extent. I can't help but think another worse demon is coming due to our collective cowardice and rejection of truth during the plandemic.

The great storm is upon us as we sail, and Jesus, it appears, is sleeping. But if you jump ship, you will die. If you are not yet in the boat, you will also perish. The storm is the rise of Antichrist, along with the Antichurch within the Church, the mystical body of the devil in the midst of the mystical body of Christ, which is already now being manifest and separating itself from the remnant of the faithful to Christ. Get into the boat, which is the Catholic Church, the Arc of Salvation. Christ is still her Captain, regardless of the treason of her first mates, for he is allowing Judases to rule His Church for reasons, I think, that have to do with the fact that we are in the end times and the Great Chastisement is imminent. And if you need any assistance to get in the boat, ask the Blessed Mother, the Arc who carried God, for it is she who crushes the head of Satan, who is terrified of and powerless against her.

Why not Untruth?

I mean, it *is* a live option. We can know something to be true, and at the same time act like it isn't, can we not? We can accept two opposing claims to be true, if we just *want* to. Nobody is stopping anyone. We can believe something knowing it's not true, sort of, or disbelieve something knowing it to be true, to some extent. In short, we can disobey truth and we can obey untruth. We *can* do it. So, why not do it? Nietzsche wondered about this, specifically, why truth was privileged and deemed a non-negotiable and exclusive starting point in thinking and discourse. This was the case for his late-nineteenth-century Germans, and further back, since the time of Plato, when the latter invented the fateful and, for Nietzsche, foolish and servile and emasculating and dishonest distinction between appearance and reality, between the shadows of untruth and the Sun of truth, between the Good and what only appears to us as such. Nietzsche:

> The Will to Truth, which is to tempt us to many a hazardous enterprise, the famous Truthfulness of which all philosophers have hitherto spoken with respect, what questions has

this Will to Truth not laid before us! What strange, perplexing, questionable questions! It is already a long story; yet it seems as if it were hardly commenced. Is it any wonder if we at last grow distrustful, lose patience, and turn impatiently away? That this Sphinx teaches us at last to ask questions ourselves? WHO is it really that puts questions to us here? WHAT really is this "Will to Truth" in us? In fact we made a long halt at the question as to the origin of this Will—until at last we came to an absolute standstill before a yet more fundamental question. We inquired about the VALUE of this Will. Granted that we want the truth: WHY NOT RATHER untruth?[23]

The obvious one-word answer to Nietzsche's question is *insanity*. Lying is knowing the truth about something but saying otherwise. The liar cares about the truth, but only for himself. But insanity is not caring about the truth at all, even for oneself. It is a sort of dedication, willing or otherwise, to untruth. To even pose the question, "Why not untruth," is to flirt with insanity, to begin walking down the path that leads to it. It is tantamount to saying, "Why not insanity," because sanity or mental health is secured and sustained through one's dedication to reality, and truth is the conformity of the mind to reality. Being dedicated to something other than and in competition with truth, then, is both an indication and cause of mental illness. M. Scott Peck:

---

[23] Friedrich Nietzsche, *Beyond Good and Evil: Prelude to a Philosophy of the Future*, trans. Helen Zimmern (New York: Dover Publications, 1997), 6.

Mental health is a dedication to reality at all costs; and mental illness occurs when the conscious will of the individual substantially deviates from the will of God, which is his or her own unconscious will. We attempt to defend our consciousness, our awareness, against reality. We do this by a variety of means which psychiatrists call defense mechanisms. All of us employ such defenses, thereby limiting our awareness. If in our laziness and fear of suffering we massively defend our awareness, then it will come to pass that our understanding of the world will bear little or no relation to reality. Although our conscious mind has denied reality, our unconscious which is omniscient, knows the true score and attempts to help us out by stimulating, through symptom formation, our conscious mind to the awareness that something is wrong. In other words, the painful and unwanted symptoms of mental illness are manifestations of grace. They are products of a powerful force, originating outside the consciousness which nurtures our spiritual growth.[24]

Nietzsche was the first philosopher to pose seriously the question, "Why not untruth," and to be taken seriously as a philosopher for doing so. The fact that he eventually went insane and never recovered is suggestive. Hamlet's question, "To be or not to be?" is an equivalent interrogative sign of imminent insanity. Your and my existence is a gift we did not give ourselves, and it is one that we can't

[24] M. Scott Peck, *The Road Less Traveled: A New Psychology of Love, Traditional Values and Spiritual Growth* (New York: Simon & Schuster, 1978), 281.

unreceive. It simply is. There was once a "not to be" for us before we existed, but not after. To pose the possibility of "not being" as if we could make this possibility a reality is to move into unreality, mental illness, insanity. What prevents the vast majority of people from seriously entertaining this question, and living it out is the loving grace of God, keeping us in reality by making us suffer pain when we depart from it, like the pain we receive from touching a hot stove from which our mother may choose one time not to protect us so the lesson is firmly learned, never to be forgotten. We all depart from reality, particularly moral reality, from time to time and to some extent whenever we choose a lesser good over a higher good, when we lie or believe a lie knowing it's a lie, when we seek to gain unjustly, when we act self-interestedly when duty-bound to care for another, etc. Internally, we suffer interior guilt for such actions, and if we repeatedly ignore or repress or rationalize the guilt, we suffer some level of mental illness. Externally, we suffer the moral opprobrium of friends and society when we trespass against the law and moral norms and customs. If we rebel against and resent this external pressure and punishment, we may be put in jail or otherwise ostracized by family, friends, and society at large. All this pain and suffering is, as Peck says, for our spiritual growth: "God chastises those He loves." Frank Sheed:

> Seeing God everywhere and all things upheld by Him is not a matter of sanctity, but of plain sanity, because God IS everywhere and all things are upheld by Him. What we do about it may be sanctity; but merely seeing it is sanity. To overlook God's presence is not simply to be irreligious; it is

a kind of insanity, like overlooking anything else that is actually there.[25]

Truth is the good of the intellect, and that's why Dante tells us that all those in Hell have "lost the good of the intellect." To ask, "Why not untruth" is thus to ask, "Why not evil," since truth and goodness are equivalent, as are untruth and evil. In seeking an answer to this question, one is seeking the truth, the good of one's intellect, so one cannot really ask this question honestly and earnestly. It is akin for me to claim right now, "I am not writing," as I write this sentence. "Why not untruth" is not a question posed to the intellect but an attack on the intellect, and so an attack on truth and reality. To even ask this question seriously and earnestly is to sin against the truth, against reality itself. It is thus to dedicate oneself to unreality, which is the definition of insanity, more specifically, moral and spiritual insanity. One would hope that, internally, God, working through what Peck calls the omniscient unconscious or what is more plainly called guilt, and, externally, society and culture through its laws, norms, customs, and other pressures and coercive punishments, will inflict enough merciful and just pain on those who are tempted to ask this question and thus dedicate themselves to unreality to prevent them from doing so, and on those who have already gone down this path, to wake them up to repentance and metanoia.

But what if not just a few insane weirdos but a whole population were to ask this anti-question, being seduced into doing so by a corrupt education and culture, and even brainwashed into doing so by trauma-based mind control, terror-ritual induced scapegoating, and

---

[25] Frank Sheed, *Theology and Sanity* (New York: Sheed & Ward, 1946), 24.

mass formation? And what if the cultural elites and their toadies were relentlessly and ubiquitously to promote and endorse and celebrate such questioning, denigrating, punishing, and marginalizing those who don't or won't ask it? This, of course, is not hypothetical. The internal defense mechanisms that usually protect the soul against consistently acting against reality are completely corrupted now, as the psychopaths who have no such internal guides have created a global pathocracy in their own image. Every institution from medicine to academia to journalism to politics is now fully predatorial and tyrannical, serving only itself and the elites at the expense of the good of those it is supposed to serve. It's worse than this. These institutions are now systematically intended to maim, paralyze, and kill, physically and spiritually, and feed off those who remain, keeping them barely alive. Everything is vampiric and parasitic now. Add to this the psychological damage of incessant propaganda rendering unreality as reality in perception and imagination, the intellectual damage of ideological indoctrination replacing liberal education and common sense and tradition, the moral damage of immersion in a culture in rebellion against the Tao, particularly in sexual matters, and the spiritual damage of a Church in apostasy, with its archleader baptizing deadly injections as sacraments of the love of neighbor, destroying by deliberate confusion the salvific doctrines and sacraments of the Faith, and offering up the Mystical Body of Christ to the globalist Luciferians, such as Schwab and Gates, to use as they see fit. In reaction to this evil, we now have self-serving Catholic "traditionalists" doing evil in the name of Catholic Tradition by rejecting completely the authority of the post-Vatican II Church and in doing so calling what is obviously holy and good, diabolical and evil. Not to mention the hordes of treasonous leftist Marxist intellectuals, who identify as Catholic but are nothing but white-washed tombs of hypocrisy and filth, serving as willing mouthpieces and maskers of the Luciferian Great Reset propaganda, from the LGBTQ agenda of normalizing pedophilia to the plandemic agenda of mass brainwashing and medical and financial enslavement, to the "sustainable development" agenda of .00001 propertied and 99.9999 (of whoever is left after they attempt to reduce the world population to 500 million) propertyless.

How is the ordinary twenty-first-century secular person, neither God-fearing, well-catechized, liberally educated, nor virtuous, supposed to save his soul, let alone remain immune from these evils and avoid the temptation to commit his life to untruth? All the rewards and blandishments are there for the taking if you do, and hell is unleashed upon you if you don't. Insane people have always considered themselves the sane ones, and psychopaths see their elite club as the superior breed, but they did not get to impose their judgments on the sane and the moral. Now they do, and they have. The insane question in Nietzsche's day was "Why not untruth?" because truth was the default existential position. The fact that Nietzsche even received a public hearing for his question indicates that things then were not good. And soon after that, the question would lose all its shock value. But it took a century and a half for untruth to become the default and only position, with even the spark of consciousness of any alternative extinguished in the collective consciousness. The result of Nietzsche's question eventually infecting the consciousness of mankind, plus a global propaganda campaign made possible by a level of technology and malice never before seen in human history, has not only been the global reign of untruth, but the spiritual lobot-omization of the masses such that the question of truth, let alone it's unimpeachable and nonnegotiable authority, is no longer posed. We all seem to be in Plato's Cave now, but without anyone to break our chains.

But God is here, and He knows what's happening, and He is al-lowing it. He can stop it in a nanosecond. But He needs to test us, and this is the final exam. He is asking, "Do you love me" every time we are confronted with propaganda, every time we are pressured to act against truth, every time we have a choice to act to gain the praise of others at the expense of our integrity and what we know to be true, every time we are tempted to ignore the warnings of others, to accept a narrative before assessing it because it makes our lives more comfortable to believe and promote it, to indulge in the self-right-eousness of scapegoating. For, to put anything, however "necessary" or "prudent" or "caring," or "progressive," above the truth in our thought and speech, and above the spiritual good of others and our-selves in our actions, is to tell Jesus that you do not love Him, and he takes our answer quite seriously. We can tell Jesus we love him, and perhaps that's all we can do at this time. I think it's good enough.

> Our life remains
> A process of guilt and obfuscation
> And it stays the same
> No closer to the deeper truths
> And further from a divine light
> We rode on wings, baring our souls / Into the night
> Leaving scattered remnants of self / When the stars fall

We fell from the sky / The depths went black

And with a blink / The lesser wind

Stood and teetered on the chasm's brink / Submitting to

the darkness

And grey, and black and nothingness

We form a line, from there to here

Hoping to find our way back.[26]

There is no power relation without the correlative constitu-

tion of a field of knowledge, nor any knowledge that does not

presuppose and constitute at the same time power rela-

tions"... it's my hypothesis that the individual is not a pre-

given entity which is seized on by the exercise of power. The

individual, with his identity and characteristics, is the prod-

uct of a relation of power exercised over bodies, multiplici-

ties, movements, desires, forces.[27]

Like Nietzsche, Michele Foucault was committed to the "truth"
that discourse is nothing but the surreptitiously coercive use of
power, and the more hidden the power, the more effective the coercion. The power hiding behind claims to truth is so all-pervasive and
effective that the very person who speaks and listens to discourse is
itself its product and mouthpiece. The conviction that I am an indi-

---

[26] Minsk, "Within and Without,' *The Crash and the Draw*, Relapse Records,
2015.

[27] Michel Foucault, *Discipline and Punish: The Birth of the Prison*, trans. Alan
Sheridan (New York: Pantheon Books, 1977), 27. "The Subject and Power," *Critical Inquiry* 8, no. 4 (Summer 1982): 777.

vidual person with agency, freedom, and knowledge before I am influenced by words and the power hiding behind them is itself a mask of power, as is the "individual" himself.

Nevertheless, Foucault used his non-agency over several decades to expose the powers hiding behind discourse systems and working to fight them. What if he had won? To replace them with what? The truth? But there is no such thing—-it's only power. Foucault was right, though, if we confine his claim to discourse, and the institutions, society, and culture in which it is exercised, *that has been thoroughly corrupted.* For, the pure purpose of words is to discover and communicate reality, whether in a declarative, optative, interrogative, or exclamatory mode, as an act of love of God and neighbor, with self-effacing worship being the highest form of speech. When words are used against their pure purpose, such as to communicate unreality to gain power over another, this is the corruption of words, and when it becomes habitual and institutionalized, it evinces precisely the characteristics Foucault describes. Josef Pieper:

Whoever speaks to another person--not simply, we presume, in spontaneous conversation but using well-considered words, and whoever in so doing is explicitly not committed to the truth-—whoever, in other words, is in this guided by something other than the truth—such a person, from that moment on, no longer considers the other as partner, as equal. In fact, he no longer respects the other as a human person. From that moment on, to be precise, all conversation ceases; all dialogue and all communication come to an end.

Public discourse, the moment it becomes basically neutralized with regard to a strict standard of truth, stands by its
nature ready to serve as an instrument in the hands of any
ruler to pursue all kinds of power schemes.[28]

2020 was the inauguration of the global institutionalization of
the corruption of discourse. Domestic terrorism by the government
(shutting down businesses, imprisoning the healthy, imposing the
wearing of oxygen-depleting masks, etc.) and the deliberate democide of the world's population through a mandatory poison injection
were successfully translated into the discourse of "public health."
And in case there were still some leftover non-corrupted elements
of discourse lying around, as well as to reinforce the mass corruption
to irreversible levels, in 2022 they held the second inauguration in
Ukraine, wherein supporting a literal Nazi genocide of Russian-
speaking Ukrainians was successfully translated into "fighting for
freedom." In 2024, the "October 7 Holocaust," in truth, an Israeli
false-flag psy-op, gave Israel and the US carte blanch authority to
commit a genocide of Palestinians. In the meantime, self-mutilation
became gender-freedom, conditioning children to tolerate and even
desire being molested, inclusive curriculum, and let's not forget the
less-recent transformation of child-murder into reproductive health
and elderly-murder into death with dignity.

The global program of discourse corruption was a top-down
agenda, orchestrated by the elites of technology, corporations, intelligence, media, finance, medicine, science, academia, as well as the

---

[28] Josef Pieper, *Abuse of Language, Abuse of Power*, trans. Lothar Krauth (San
Francisco: Ignatius Press, 1992), 21.

various alphabet-soup agencies of global control (WEF, NIH, CIA, WHO, FDA, CDC, etc.), the multitude of satanic foundations and thinktanks (Rockefeller, Council on Foreign Relations), and let's not leave out the City of London, the Zionists, and the Freemasons. But it couldn't have been as successful as it was without the cooperation of first the lower-tier rulers of discourse in the professions, business, religion, the arts, entertainment, education, tech industry, media, government bureaucracy, and management, and then the rest of us ordinary people, who used to be called the unwashed masses, but should now be called the brainwashed masses.

I am not writing this for the psychopaths and those confirmed in wickedness at the source of this malevolent fountain of language corruption, the die-hard Foucaultians in theory and practice. And I am not writing for their lower-tier cooperators, those whose talents and vocations have put them in positions of cultural influence, but whose cowardice, venality, vanity, spite, envy, sloth, hypocrisy, virtue-signaling, faux-compassion, ambition, and overall worldliness has led them to complicity in deception and slander for what they can get personally and career-wise. In Catholic circles, these types are legion on both the "right," neocons, and the "left," progressives—what binds them together is their worship of state power. These are so immersed in the corrupt discourse and so good at making the best of it that they wouldn't know how to live outside of it, and they don't want to.

Rather, I am writing to and for those of you aware of this corruption, for the most part at least, and are more victims than agents of this corruption, but who, due to the power and subtleness of this corruption, could too easily become agents—it is to help us avoid both victimage and complicity and to empower us to unmask and destroy the corruption, that I write. If you are still reading this, then it means that you hate the supreme evil of using language to manipulate and gain power, and would rather die than commit it. The first thing I want to say is that if you are indeed committed to using language as God intended it to be used, as an instrument of love, in the present climate, and it's only getting worse, you are going to be hated, persecuted, gaslighted, mocked, canceled, scapegoated, driven to insanity (if you let them), and, in the not too distant future, murdered—many of those most dangerous to the lie-regime have indeed been murdered since the Plandemic began. But it seems to me that the violence will eventually spread to anyone committed to the truth and unwilling to hide this commitment.

The second important thing is that though we have this commitment to truth above power, the corruption is so pervasive and insidious that we are inevitably tainted with it, meaning that there are beliefs and judgments we are used to holding and asserting as true that are actually just vectors of power relations put into our minds by hidden manipulation and brainwashing. What those are in particular are for you to discover, but they are there. Pray and be quiet, watch and observe, inquire and doubt, read outside your comfort zone, accept the suffering of cognitive dissonance and the loss of some social relations and worldly securities that will come when you recognize and renounce what Pierre Grimes has called the *pathologoi* in your soul.[29]

---

[29] Pierre Grimes and Regina L. Uliana, *Philosophical Midwifery: A New Paradigm for Understanding Human Problems With Its Validation* (Huntington Beach, CA: Hyparxis Press, 1990).

Thirdly, it is imperative to find others to talk to and be with who are committed to truth over power, and I mean actually committed, not just claiming to be or having the standard beliefs of someone who is committed It's hard to find the good souls, but if they are present to you when you talk to them, and you really feel their presence, and if they are willing to suffer for you, when no one is looking, that's some sure signs of their commitment. Finally, take heart in the fact that God loves and protects those who refuse to put power over truth, because this means you desire Heaven, and His will, approval, and presence, more than anything else, and this makes Him happy.

What has been Revealed

Medicine, science, technology, academia, law, politics, economics, journalism,—these and all the sundry institutions of contemporary, western, secular liberal society and culture are now in a state of complete corruption. And I mean *complete*. Incomplete corruption entails intact ends, but corrupt means, e.g., medicine seeking to promote health, but, due to greed or incompetence, promoting illness instead. Complete corruption ensues when the natural ends themselves are no longer sought.

Medicine, instead of promoting health and life, now promotes illness and death—consider the poisonous and deadly spikeshot that called itself a vaccine. Science, instead of promoting empirical truth based upon impartial research, now peddles empirical falsehoods based upon ideology. Technology, instead of helping man to harness nature for his flourishing, now works to enslave the many to the few. Academia, far from being a bastion of free inquiry ordered to truth, now is nothing but woke group-think ordered to power. Journalism reports lies as truth, politics secures the common evil, economics destroys wealth, and media mediates unreality.

What's the reason for this systemic and absolute corruption? Did a group of evil, psychopathic men infiltrate these institutions and get into positions of power? Well, yes, certainly. But the question remains as to how and why *that* happened. My thesis is that absolute corruption is what happens and what must happen when societal institutions are officially divorced from natural and supernatural reality, when they are set up and made to function as self-sufficient entities, needing no explicit, corporate, and deliberate grounding in the true and the good. When man, a creature of God, acts as if he were self-created and independent, he becomes a monster. It is the same with institutions. First, they are corrupted by atheist ideology (whether explicit as in Marxism or cloaked as in Liberalism), then they are taken over by psychopaths and their wicked minions.

I have been committed to this thesis on an intellectual level for some time now, but it is something else to see its truth playing out in practice right before our eyes. Ever since I figured this out decades ago, after reading Plato's *Republic,* Christopher Dawson, and the Encyclicals of Leo XIII, I have been trying to help people, especially Catholic academics, to see this truth, at least on an intellectual level in terms of logic, of what follows and must follow from first principles, the primary of which being that politics flows from culture, culture from religion, and religion from theology. But now, the truth is right here in living color, manifest, concrete, palpable, in front of our eyes. The incarnate revelation of evil.

I had once thought that when the obviously evil consequences of diabolically evil ideas, such as the grotesque, cunningly hidden god-lessness of liberalism, became manifest in existential and material reality, the masses would wake up, repent, revolt, overthrow the elite of psychopaths and Luciferians in power, and work with the grace of God to establish a new Christendom. Well, the evil consequences are here now in spades—virtually the entire global population in-jected itself with a deadly, human-genome-altering poison, and the leaders of the Church that the God-Man Himself founded promoted this diabolical sorcery—and I see no sign of such a graced response, though there have been pockets of resistance. Quite the contrary. It is as if the whole world was under diabolical possession. And now it is in remission—for a time. The end game is the voluntary, consen-sual spiritual self-enslavement of every human being to the will of Satan via a technocratic globalist elite. The means to this is staged "crises" (fake pandemics, false-flag provoked wars) that tempt us to turn on our own brothers and sisters and cry out to the minions of antichrist for salvation from the very evils they have caused.

God allowed these demonic elites to torture us so that their masks fall off and we finally realize that rejecting God as our Father, we don't get to govern ourselves, as liberalism tells us. The only al-ternative to submission to the Living God who gave His Blood for us is enslavement to vampiric monsters who lust for our blood. God is allowing this final chastisement—and it is going to get worse—so that so that as many people as possible will recognize Him, cry out to Him, and repent. God cares about nothing more than the salva-tion of souls. We are His creatures, and we are to obey and live in His will. He has given us the gift to do this on earth. It is the same

with the institutions that we have created in modern times. They are
to be instruments of His will, ordered and grounded in it, not instruments of human will in rebellion against reality and thus His will,
the ground of reality. There is no neutrality, no "secular," no "liberal," no "separation of Church and state." There is just the Holy
Will of God, and all humans and human institutions must be obedi-
ent to it. If they are not, they have hell to pay, both now and in eternity. And this is also a consequence of God's love. He will bring us
into His arms, even if it's because the only alternative is the hideous
mouth of the devil.

Silence, long held
in shuttered cities
Landscape pocked with bodies
Stale breath hovers
Piled high under common eye
the naked dead flow
A stream uninterrupted
in light of day
Rats stir, quiver
under sun's unbidden pallor
Oh, muted hearts
through clasped hands glimmer
Shine!
Hearts! Shine!
Steps falter
in halls long emptied
Dull gaze glistens

through shadowed cracks
Mask broken
Blood, across all shores
twined
By the fall
all are joined
Through red cloud's haze
finger's reach is met
All are joined
All are joined
Sight regained
In rooms now illumed
by fire's shine
Swaying mass
by hymns restored
Up the luminous steps
Arisen from the ash they ascend
Up! Up!
Ascend!
By shards of sun scattered
Through dome hung with leaves
are anointed bowed heads
In this world of light.[30]

There are two ways to discern the Will of God for one's life. One is to discover what God has revealed about it in His own words, and this is to be found in Catholicism, with no admixture of error. By

---

[30] Sumac, *"World of Light,"* track 5 on *The Healer,* Thrill Jockey Records, 2024,

practicing it, one is also enabled to believe with certainty and follow with consistency what God has revealed through Grace, the theological virtues of Faith, Hope, and Charity that are infused into the soul in Baptism, through participation in the sacraments, and a life of prayer, contemplation, and grace-inspired, meritorious, loving works. While Faith provides access to the supernatural aspect of God's Will, undiscoverable and incomprehensible to the human intellect, His will can also be known on a natural level in creation through the exercise of theoretical and practical reason. For example, what God wants us to do is communicated through the moral law, which is discernible by reason alone. And the acquired virtue of prudence, aided by the infused virtue of the prudence and the Holy Spirit's gift of counsel, indeed, by all of the acquired and infused virtues and gifts, allows one to discern God's will in the immanent particulars of one's daily life.

There is a lot more I could say about this way of knowing God's Will, including the role that liberal education and familial/political/cultural habituation play in disposing us to see it and love it, not to mention the conditioning influence of one's political and cultural order, healthy or corrupt or somewhere in between, and the present condition of the human element of the Church, with its relation to the political and cultural, whether subservient or authoritative or somewhere in between. Regardless of these factors and conditions, everything every human being has ever and will ever need to discern the Will of God and obey It is available, for God desires that all men be saved and come to the knowledge of the Truth, and thus He provides to every human being at every moment in every place what is necessary to obtain salvation, if we so desire it, choose it, and cooperate with His abundant Grace. Desiring it and choosing it is up to us, for God who created us without our will will not save us without it.

But there is another way to discern the Will of God, not through what God has directly revealed about Himself and His Will, but through what God has permitted His enemies to reveal in their opposition to Him. In addition to the first way, and for many it is now the main path to it, it is this "negative" revelation of God's will that God wants us to turn our attention to, whether we have the Catholic Faith or not. Just as God allows heresies to arise so that the full and balanced truth can be more deeply and accurately understood in contrast, so too is God allowing not mere heresy but an all-out assault of all the combined forces of evil on God, His Church, and Reality itself, both from within the Church and without, so that we can more fully and deeply understand the saving truths and realities in which we may already believe and experience to be exquisitely prepared to do His Will in the present time.

If everything needed for salvation is present to us, and guaranteed to be such, for against the Church the Gates of Hell cannot prevail; and since evil cannot prevent us from choosing to do God's will, then the only thing the forces of evil can do is to make it as difficult as possible to do so. God allows them to make it so difficult, and we wish He did not, and we cannot really explain why He does so. We only know that it's somehow better for us this way. When we look back on our lives from Heaven, we will have more understanding of this, but until then, we must simply trust and submit to His all-loving and all-merciful and all-just and knowing and all-powerful will.

So what is evil doing right now to make things as difficult as possible, and what can we learn from it so as to defeat it? This is the topic of the next chapter.

Chapter III

The Victory

Weaponized Truths

The New World Order that has emerged from and through the plandemic, a Dis-Order of technocratic, totalitarian rule, a globalist hunger-games economy of hundreds of masters and billions of slaves, and incessant and endless trauma-based mind control and terrorism, must be resisted at all costs, for it is the attempt to set up an antichrist system based upon a complete rejection of God, the Church, and reality. To fight this, we need first principles and grounding truths, the fundamental truths of *logos*, the metaphysical, moral, and spiritual order of the universe, accessible to human reason and perfected in the Divine Revelation of Jesus Christ. These comprise an indispensable bulwark and shield against the enemies of reality that are now engaged in an all-scale attack on human life. And we need to weaponize these truths and go to battle.

Spiritual/Theological Truths:

1. The universe did not make itself, as it is not a necessary being. Thus, it must have been the creation of an omnipotent, omniscient, eternal God. Indeed, reality itself is continually being created and sustained in existence, moment-by-moment, by this God, who, being perfect, is infinite love and perfect happiness. Every moment,

event, and circumstance of our lives is an ongoing gift of this God to us out of his infinite gratuitousness.

If we knew this, we would never fall into idolatry, never expect from man and nature what can only come from God and super-nature. And we would have a formidable spiritual and psychological strength born of trust in both God's power, goodness, and providential intimacy. We would never adopt a servile fear of God's enemies but boldly stand against them, encouraging others to do the same, knowing that God wins and evil loses, always and everywhere.

2. God created human beings in His divine image to know, love, and serve Him because in doing so we participate and share in His infinite divinity and perfect happiness, and His loving will for every human being He has created is to share in His Divinity. Since God is eternal, such participation for us means eternal life with and in Him, beginning now and continuing forever after we die.

If we knew this, we would never fall into worldliness and idola-trous attachments, which are the hooks with which evil men keep us enslaved. We would never be willing to do anything that would jeop-ardize our salvation, such as putting loyalty to truth second to worldly advantage, the treason that so many Christians committed in 2020.

3. We cannot know, love, and serve Him without His assistance because we are born with an ineradicable tendency to selfishness, separateness, and disobedience, rooted in pride and ignorance. Thus, prayer in all its forms—vocal, mental, meditative, silent, com-munal, liturgical—through which we access this assistance, is the most important and essential human activity.

If we knew this, we would never allow the simulacrum of the technocracy to distract us and drown out the silence in which we commune with God. We would become walking liturgies in which others detect the presence of God. By making prayer the primary activity of our daily lives, our very being, apart from any good works we do, will radiate God's power and love, defeating his enemies before a word is spoken or action taken.

4. Knowledge and love of God make us like Him, and since He is love itself, love of neighbor flows inevitably from our growing likeness to Him. If we are not loving our neighbor to the best of our ability, it means we are rejecting our likeness to God and our creaturely obligation.

We have enemies. The Church has enemies. Ancient and ineradicable and relentless and implacable enemies. Our neighbor may be our enemy. But we identify them, call them out, and love them, precisely because they are our enemies. The neo-pagan alt-righters accurately identify the enemies of Western civilization and the moral law, but because they see Christianity as an enemy, they hate these enemies. We love our enemies, and in doing so, which may include harsh rebuke and just discrimination, we defeat them with love and lead many of them to conversion. If we know this truth, we also love our neighbors who are not our enemies, and we do so as we reject a tribal, inner-circle, gnostic neo-pharisaism, which is not of Christ but of the Devil. Catholic traditionalists take heed.

5. Both human reason and Divine Faith allow every human being to recognize Jesus Christ as the only possible human incarnation of the God described above.

The global antichrist religion that has emerged and gained much influence and power as I write this is at its core syncretistic. It would have us believe in Jesus Christ, but not as the only and definitive expression of God on earth, with the Catholic Church as His only mystical body on earth, outside of which there is no salvation. This just won't do in the twenty-first century. Many Catholics will fall for the Antichrist precisely because of his surreptitious and implicit denial of the Incarnation, which will seem much more reasonable, enlightened, charitable, and tolerant than that old, fundamentalist, and narrow Catholicism, one that, after all, as every good modern person knows, has caused so much bloodshed, division, and hatred throughout history.

Metaphysical Truths

1. All that exists is good because being itself is good, as well as true and beautiful.

2. The universe as a whole, as well as every part of it, is purposeful and intelligent, being made by a purposeful and intelligent creator.

3. Evil exists, but it is parasitical—it has no independent being. It is a real absence of a real good that should exist but doesn't due to deliberately bad human choices.

We are now experiencing a level and ubiquity of evil unprecedented in the history of the world. It might seem from that evil is competing with good, and winning. We may be tempted to take the black pill and lose our hope and innocence. Has not evil taken control of not only the world but also the Church? What could be eviler than the holder of the office of St. Peter obligating billions of Catholics under penalty of being "unloving" to be injected with what is now known to be a bioweapon[1] as part of a satanic program of global terrorism and democide, on the one hand, and requiring Catholic priests to bless sodomite couples, on the other? Hasn't evil shown itself to be in charge? Hasn't goodness been shown to be a naïve myth, a childish fairy tale? If we know the metaphysical truths about goodness and evil, we will never fall into despair. God is in charge and has already won, and evil, no matter how gruesome and inexplicable and insufferable, is deliberately permitted by God for our good, for the greatest good. This is the truth. You must know it and never doubt it.

4. Human beings can become evil in their souls due to deliberate, knowing, choices against the Good and their morally informed consciences. If they persist in these choices and do not repent of them, they will be punished for them in both this and the next life.

Yes, evil is just an absence of being, a parasite, but, still, there are evil people. Malicious people. People who do evil knowing that it is evil and for the sake of evil. No, not everyone is "just trying to do the right thing." This is nothing but a cowardly and sentimental refusal to acknowledge the obvious. Malice exists. And this is why Hell exists, and why it is eternal, for people can choose evil in their last earthly moments, and Hell is what they choose. They would have it no other way. If we understand this truth, we will have an accurate understanding of the people who are ruling us and their evil agenda.

---

[1] See the work of Katherine Watt: https://bailiwicknews.substack.com/p/american-domestic-bioterrorism-program.

Mistakes were not made in 2020[2]—they intended to torture, enslave, and murder us, and they still do, and not because they "think it is good." They know it is evil, and that is why they do it. They are Satanists.

5. Reality is more than mere matter, for it includes immutable, immaterial substantial form and eternal spirit. Matter doesn't exist without the unchanging form that gives it definite essence and existence. And form doesn't exist without matter, without some level of potency, as in the angels, which are immaterial but not without potency, potency toward existence. Only God is pure actuality.

6. Human beings are comprised of matter, form, and spirit, or, using different terms, body and soul. We are neither souls nor bodies alone, but soul and body syntheses or composites.

7. Death is the separation of our body and soul, but since the soul is one and indivisible, it is immortal.

Angelism, denying matter, and materialism, denying form, are the errors this truth vanquishes. Both are the errors of modernity. Technocracy and the digitalization of everything deny both the limiting existence of matter and the inexorable givenness of form, while godless hedonism, consumerism, therapeuticism, and the secularization and sexualization of culture and politics deny spirit. Well-being, not salvation, is the primary desideratum behind these errors, and hell on earth and after it is the result. If we understand these metaphysical truths, we will pursue salvation over well-being, and well-being only for the sake of salvation.

---

[2] Margaret Anna Alice, "Mistakes Were NOT Made: An Anthem," *Margaret Anna Alice Through the Looking Glass*, Substack, accessed January 1, 2025, https://margaretannaalice.substack.com/p/mistakes-were-not-made-an-anthem.

8. All men by nature desire to know, and for the sake of knowing, since it is in knowing, loving, and acting in accordance with the Truth that men find their perfection and happiness.

This truth is a shield against:

- evolutionism/radical existentialism, which claims that men do not share a common nature, or if they do, it's merely a biological adaption subject to further change.
- utilitarianism/pragmatism, which claims that men may desire to know, but only as a means to the useful or pleasurable.

9. The human intellect can distinguish between what appears, on the one hand, and what *is,* on the other, that is, between opinion and knowledge. Thus, Truth exists and can be known as such, but we must recognize the limits and mode of human knowing, both tradition-dependent and tradition-transcendent.

This is a shield against:

- relativism/skepticism, which claims that knowledge is subjective and relative.
- Kantianism/empiricism, which claims that our experience is never of what is, but only of what appears.
- rationalism/Cartesian idealism/angelism/gnosticism, which claims that both objective truth and the human mode of knowing are absolute.
- postmodernism, which claims that both reality and human rationality are subjective and relative. There is only discourse and narratives, never objective truth.

10. Truth is the conformity of our minds to reality (through human reason), and our minds to the mind of God (through prayer and the gift of Faith).

This is a shield against:

- empiricism/idealism, which claims that truth is the conformity of our statements to our sense-impressions or ideas.
- materialism, which claims that while truth is the conformity of our mind to reality, the real is merely material.
- deconstructionism/Nietzschean nihilism, which claims that truth is only the mask of power.
- naturalism/modernism, which claims that we cannot know the mind of God, only our own minds.

11. All human actions are determined by thought and will (practical reason), which is the conformity of the intellect to the truth about the Good, and conformity of rational desire (the will) to right reason.

This is a shield against:

- voluntarism/existentialism/sentimentalism, which claims that human actions are determined either by will or desire alone, not reason.
- determinism/behaviorism, which claims that human thought and action are determined by culture, upbringing, or genetics.

12. We are obliged by natural law to love and do good and to hate and avoid evil, and therefore we must be able to know the difference between good and evil, objectively and absolutely.

This is a shield against:

- voluntarism, which claims that the only authoritative law and norm of goodness or evil is God's will as revealed in Scripture and the Church.
- historicism/moral relativism, which claims that what is considered good is not based in absolute and unchangeable reality but relative to person, culture, or history.
- Kantian deontology, which claims that while morality is objective and absolute, it is so because it derives from our own minds, which are absolute, not nature or God.

13. The human intellect can grasp universal truth, and it can know essences and the causes of things.

This is a shield against:

- Kantianism/nominalism, which claims that the universals are only in the mind, not in things.
- extreme Platonism, which claims that the universals exist only as forms in a transcendent realm completely separate from existing things.

14. The attainment of Wisdom, not power or pleasure, is the purpose of our knowing. Wisdom is the loving knowledge of the

most important truths about God and the universe accompanied by
an inclination of the will to live and act in accordance with them.

This is a shield against:

- Straussianism, which claims that the purpose of philosophical study is endless questioning with no absolute truth discoverable.
- intellectualism/Phariseeism/gnosticism, which claims that the purpose of study is knowledge to gain spiritual power.
- pragmatism/hedonism/Baconianism/therapeuticism, which claims that the purpose of study is pleasure, well-being, or worldly power.

15. Knowing and loving in the natural, created order should prepare and dispose the mind for supernatural, mystical knowing and loving in supernatural, divine order.

This is a shield against:

- fideism/naturalism, which claims that Faith and reason are incompatible.
- pantheism/monism/supernaturalism, which claims that there is no "nature"—all is God, all is supernatural.
- eastern/new-age/kabbalistic irrationalism, which claims that mysticism is the highest knowledge, but it is incompatible with philosophy or human reason, and material and moral reality.

Moral and Political Truths

1. The human person is inherently good; therefore, he must never be treated by other humans as a means but only as an end.

2. Men are social and political animals; thus, they find their perfection and happiness and good with each other in political community.

3. The purpose of political community is to secure the material, moral, and spiritual conditions in which human beings can thrive and flourish, and humans thrive and flourish together through virtuous activity and contemplation of God.

4. The natural law, which is the set of moral laws that govern the universe ordered to human good, happiness and perfection, is a higher authority than the political law, and thus both leaders and citizens must act in accordance with it as its subjects.

5. Since human laws must be ordered to the human good and be in accordance with the natural law, when they are not, citizens are under no obligation to obey them.

6. Just as human persons owe in justice obedience to and worship of God, so too do human persons in community, including the political community; thus, a godless political community is unjust and evil.

7. If the political community, with its laws, institutions, economic structures, and cultural norms, is not ordered to the natural law and God, it will necessarily become tyrannical

and totalitarian, for it will exalt man's will over God's will, human law over the natural law, and lies over truth.

We are now living under global totalitarianism precisely because of the denial of the preceding truths and the institutionalization of this denial. Jesus told us that the Devil is a liar and a murderer from the beginning. There is nothing more evil than lying and murdering, no straighter path to Hell than the one paved by them, and never before has there been more lies and murders. Geo-politically, the plandemic was an onslaught of lies and murder, with the false-flag terror event of IXXI its prelude. The War on Terror that IXXI inaugurated, which destroyed so many countries and lives and ushered in the first stage of global totalitarianism, was built on an enormous lie, and if the reader doesn't know this, that's just indicative of how powerful the lie was. The number of deaths from the bioweapon injection is already in the tens of millions, not to mention the incalculable amount of physical and psychological sickness it and the psy-op as a whole unleashed, and the death toll may very well rise to a billion in the next few years, considering that we still do not know what exactly they put in the jabs and why they were so intent on jabbing everyone on the planet, not to mention the potential for harm of the nanotech and graphene oxide that we know were in them. Everything, literally everything, they told us in 2020 and after was a lie, and these lies were aimed at the total subjugation of society and human souls. They were incredibly successful. And they are creating new and bigger lies every day, and doubling down on the previous ones.

The Devil cannot force us to lie or murder, only tempt us to do so, but what he can do is use his willing servants to create lies and then force us to live in the midst of them. He's been doing this since the foundation of the world, beginning with the First Lie through the willing serpent: "You shall not die. You shall be as gods knowing good and evil." But he had to wait until the 21st century, with its centralized, elite-controlled, technologically advanced media, to create lies that could become literal worlds, with his minions forcing the rest of us to inhabit them. This he has done. We can't entirely escape these worlds, but we can recognize the lies upon which they are built, resist them, reject them in our own minds and hearts, unmask them for all to see, substitute them with truths, and weaponize them. But how many are doing this? How many of those with some power and influence in society are doing so? How many Christians are doing so? How many Catholics?

What the Devil wants most is for us to become complicit with and participate in these lie worlds, not necessarily by creating them in the first place (this is the special prerogative of the evilest among), or by believing in them wholeheartedly and earnestly (for this can be done without sin, with all or most of the fault and guilt in the liar and not the lied-to, with the main fault of the latter being, not dishonesty, but mere stupidity and gullibility), but in accepting them while not really believing in them, or without putting in the effort to question and determine their truth, preferring instead to live within and promote these lie-worlds instead of the real world due to the enhancement of one's power, sense of well-being, prestige, etc. that the public acceptance and parroting of them secures. One knows in

the back of one's mind that the claims and narratives are either untrue or not indubitably the truth, but one still speaks and behaves as
if they are self-evident, unquestionable, sacred, the mere doubting
of which being indicative of insanity or malice. Doing so preserves
one's status and power in the world. One becomes a traitor to Truth.

8. The moral obligation to worship and follow God according to
our consciences, and thus the freedom to do so, is part of the natural
and divine law; thus, the State must not only do anything to hinder
the exercise of this freedom, but it should also assist citizens in fulfilling this obligation.

Christ is King. All of the preceding spiritual, theological, metaphysical, moral, and political truths could be effectively weaponized
for the good if we just had the courage to know them deeply and live
them out. We chose to live in the lie-worlds that were created, trans-
mitted, and incarnated in politics and culture insofar as we believed
in them, unaware, but perhaps not completely unaware, of their
mendacity. Many of these lie-worlds, from the most abstract and
ideological (materialism, secularism, scientism, liberalism, radical
feminism, Americanism, Zionism) to the most concrete and historical (WWII allied war crimes and propaganda, and violent deep-
state/false-flag events, such as the JFK assassination, IXXI, and the
Scamdemic) are now being contested and unmasked in the consciousness of an increasing number of people. They are now being
revealed, not as indubitable and obvious truths and facts of nature
and history, but as man-made ideologies and paradigms and egre-
gores, psyops, propaganda narratives, and Orwellian double-think,
originating in the will-to-power of ruling elites and imposed on the

collective consciousness by nefarious personages, intelligence agencies, secret societies, and globalist institutions, also being unmasked and named.

God is allowing these lies and schemes to be exposed, and we are recognizing that we have been lied to about the most fundamental things, from the nature of God and reality and political order to the "facts" of cosmology, history, and health, and many are speaking out, such as Candace Owens, who has been challenging many sacred cows in public on behalf of the masses. Dr. David Hughes is one of the very few public academics telling the full truth about the plandemic and other deep state crimes against humanity. He writes:

> A categorical refusal to believe in absurdities is, therefore, indispensable to resisting evil. It is not only an intellectual requirement, but also a moral and theological imperative. Today, the effectiveness of the Big Lie technique is waning. More and more people are refusing to believe in absurdities simply because their government and media tell them to. With this "Great Awakening" will come a powerful religious resurgence, because the lies are designed to sustain evil, while the truth allows good to flourish.[3]

With all these propaganda narratives crumbling before our eyes, will the academic class and other establishment professionals who have served as gate-keepers, either ignoring the "conspiracy theories" entirely or providing intellectual cover for them, finally repent

---

[3] David A. Hughes, "Resistance and Faith," *David A. Hughes Substack*, June 27, 2024, https://dhughes.substack.com/p/resistance-and-faith.

of their cowardice and treason, or will they all double down and become confirmed in evil? In the last five years or so, several Catholic academics, D.C. Schindler in particular, have thoroughly unmasked the Big Lie of liberalism and have publicly endorsed some form of Catholic integralism or confessionalism, which is the only rational position for a believing Catholic, thereby making it "safe" for others to do so. There was a time when this way of thinking was considered insane or heretical or wicked (think of First Things under Fr. Neuhaus) but at that time some heroic Catholic intellectuals did their job (David Schindler the Elder, God rest his soul, in particular) and now Catholic public discourse permits such thoughts. They have won the debate. But how many establishment academics are willing to use their trained intellectual powers and influential platforms to weaponize the truths they know, to call into question not just relatively safe-to-critique ideological lies but the much more dangerous, hot-button, third-rail ones, such as the deep-state, trauma-based psy-ops mentioned above that were enabled by these ideologies and now keep so many people in psychological and spiritual bondage? Thes truths also need to be weaponized, not just the abstract and relatively safe ones.

It is both the case that it's the best time ever to become a Catholic and the worst. It's the best because we are literally living through the Great Storm and Great Tribulation preceding the Warning and the arrival of the Antichrist, and due to the fact that the world has never been as evil as it is today, the amount of grace God is pouring out upon us is unprecedented. It is the time for heroic saints wielding the Sword of Truth, and who in their right mind doesn't want to be part of the most dramatic and urgent and epic battle ever to occur in the history of mankind? It's the worst time, however, because of the confusion and evil within the Church, as an antichurch emerges from hiding and the abomination of desolation attempts to occupy the holy of holies. Homosexuality and pedophilia normalization, transgenderism, global totalitarianism, and transhumanism are evils hard enough to fight with the help of the Church, but when her human element and ruling apparatus are compromised by and even complicit in these same evils, it seems impossible and hopeless.

So, let us know deeply and weaponize these truths and the Truth, in our own way and according to our particular circumstances, personal vocation, and unique inspirations from the Holy Spirit, to defeat the enemies of the Church and humanity, the enemies of all that is good, true, and beautiful, for the sake of God's glory, above all, but also for the renewal of the Church and the culture, and the salvation of souls.

The Power of Authority

Modernity is the attempt to do away with authority and replace it with power. All that is needed, modernity says, because all there is, is coercive power. And there never was authority, only power, power pretending to be authority. Authority is the mask that power once used effectively to coerce. It functioned well for a time, but since the Enlightenment, and especially after Foucault and the 20th century, its mask is off now, for we all know now that all there is is power. Victims now have all the power, or those who claim to be victims. It's better that the mask is off and gone, because just the appearance of the mask might lead one to think that authority actually exists, exists apart from power, exists even above power, and this could threaten the exclusive hegemony of power.

Religion used to exert power, but it also claimed authority, but since authority has been shown to be only power, and since religion no longer coerces, even if it tries to, religion now has no power. If it has power, it's because it no longer has authority. People do still believe in religion, but the vast majority do so no longer as an authority—that small remnant that still does is inconsequential and diminishing fast, and it will soon recognize that what it worshipped and always worshipped was power. If people still believe in the authority of religion, say, Christianity, they do so, even if they don't think and say they do, as something that gives them personal power, either in this life or in the next, or so they believe. Death, it must be admitted, takes away all power, so some believe in religion because it seems to give them power even over death. As I say, some people still attribute authority to their religion, even saying "Christ is King!" But when it comes down to it, they don't think or act much like this—or only an insignificant minority does, and they won't for too much longer, especially when Antichrist comes, whose perfect power will finally annihilate authority for good —for these always obey power, and particularly power without authority, and they defend it as such.

A good example of these truths (of course, there is no truth, only power) was the plandemic, which was the apotheosis (so far) of power without authority. Most religious people believed in it, obeyed it, and defended it as if it were an authority, one that *should* be believed, obeyed, and defended. But here's the thing. They knew it wasn't an authority. Why? Because it was nothing but coercion, and everyone knows, if they could just think about what they know for a minute, that authority doesn't coerce. For that's what authority is: non-coercive power. But they obeyed this totalitarian onslaught of coercion, and they did so without resisting it, or even questioning it. This is the crux. They treated the plandemic as an authority that should not be questioned, but they knew it was just power, because it coerced them, and coercive power should always be interrogated to see if it is authorized. They knew this, but they acted against what they knew. If power is authorized, then one should accept it and obey it. But they believed in and obeyed coercive power without questioning it, and they defended their belief and obedience as if they were defending a legitimate authority as if they were defending authorized power. They didn't just say, "I must believe and obey, but I don't want to or think I should," which is something one says when coerced by power without authority, but they said, "It is good that I believe and obey—and I want to," which is something one says to an authority, and to authorized power. Jorge Bergoglio who is believed by billions to have the authority of the Pope, even said that love obligates one to inject oneself with the Covid injection. Many religious people, the plandemic revealed, aren't religious at all, for they worship power, power *as* authority, which is to say, they reject all authority other than power, their own power above all, including the authority of Truth and God. Now that's a revelation.

So, what is authority? Well, authority, whatever it is, is not coercive. Only power is. This is difficult to grasp and must be unpacked. When Jesus Christ informed Pilate that His kingdom was not of this world, what He meant was that His Kingdom *is* Authority, not power, but *all* authority, *the* authority, eternal authority for all the exercises of temporal power from the beginning of the world until its end. But what is authority? And how does it differ from power? I will make a claim, and then I will try to answer these questions. But I am not sure if I will be able to. My claim is that Jesus Christ crucified is absolute authority combined with absolute powerlessness. And that the Jews who crucified Him had absolute power—the power to murder God—combined with an absolute absence of authority.

The Latin is *auctoritas*, from *auctor* (which also gives us English "author"), which is derived from Latin augeō ("to augment", "to enlarge", "to enrich"). If you look at any modern English definition of authority, it will define it in terms of power, always describing authority as a kind of power, namely, that power that is "justified" or "legitimate." But this is wrong, for authority is not power. And power is not authority. Authority *per se* is powerless. Jesus' authority was not recognized when He was on the cross precisely because of the profound error of thinking that any true authority always possesses and exercises power. Since Jesus was, by His own choice but also by the inexorable logic of love, powerless on the cross, it must be that He had no authority, it would seem. And this wasn't just the error of the Jews who hated Him, but even of those who loved Him, including Peter, the Prince of the Apostles, who denied knowing Him precisely because he could no longer recognize His authority when He was arrested and beaten and judged by the masses and the Roman and Jewish leaders to be guilty of evil. Since they had power, all the power at that moment, and Jesus did not, had no power at all (it seemed), it must be that they also had at least some authority and that Jesus had none. Peter did not recognize Jesus' authority, let alone his absolute divine authority as God, because Jesus at that point had no power. If He had power, He would have not allowed Himself to be tortured and crucified. How could this be denied? Whether John and the two Marys, who didn't deny knowing Jesus and remained with Him under the cross, fully recognized His authority at that moment is not clear. But they did stay with Him. They remained in the agony of knowing and not knowing, which is all they could have done. God was pleased with that.

If authority is powerless, then what is it, and how does it relate to power? For these do seem inextricably related. God, the Omnipotent One is powerless to achieve what He wants the most. What He wants most is for rational creatures to obey Him, for if they did, they would love Him for His own sake, which is what He commands, which is all He commands, with every other command being ordered to and a means to this one. For Him to achieve this, however, rational creatures must freely, without coercion, recognize His authority. He can certainly make them recognize and obey Him out of fear of punishment or desire for reward, and this was the Old Testament "classroom management" training, but this is only to recognize and obey His power, not His authority, for we are only doing so to gain some personal power of our own, the way the pagans worshipped Zeus. What He wants is something no Pagan god wanted, for us to love Him for His own sake, not for what we can get from loving Him, and this would be to recognize His authority, not His power. God has no power to make us do this, the thing He wants the most. The most He could do was to allow Himself to suffer and die for us, but the greatest suffering He felt, the Servant of God Luisa

Picarretta tells us, was in the Garden of Gethsemane when he saw all the people in Hell that He was powerless to save because they wouldn't recognize His authority, and He couldn't make them.[4]

As I try to say exactly what authority is and how it differs from power, I keep coming back to examples. I have been taking courses in a credential program so I can keep my teaching job at a public charter high school. It occurred to me recently that the methods of teaching they promote, and the only ones they recognize as authoritative, are those of power, not authority. Oh, they talk a lot about asserting your "authority" in the classroom, but what they really mean is asserting your power. This is "class management." Management is about power. The manager is a modern character, as Alasdair MacIntyre taught us, because his job is to manage power, and modernity, as we have said, is the replacement of authority with power. If things aren't managed well, the manager has failed, and he didn't have to fail because if he used his power effectively, things—or people—would have been managed well, and he could have managed his power more effectively. He just needed more training. For the State of California's educational "authority," it's the same with students. There are strategies for managing a classroom, and if you follow them, the students will be well-managed. And if you are observed for a teaching evaluation, and the students aren't all "engaged" and "on task," it means that you failed as a classroom manager, which is pretty much your only task as a teacher.

I was observed once, and the evaluation report indicated that I needed to improve in classroom management. This got me thinking

---

[4] Luisa Piccarreta, *The Hours of the Passion of Our Lord Jesus Christ*, trans. Antonio F. Borelli, 2nd ed. (Evangeline Press, 2009).

about authority and power in the classroom. I could easily have used my power to force the students, through the threat of punishment and seduction of reward, to appear engaged and on task to the observer, or even to be engaged and on task (if the task was directly related to threat or seduction), but that is not what my power as a teacher is for. The power I have as a teacher is no different than the power I have as a human being, and it is for the same ultimate purpose, to help my neighbor get to Heaven, thus to know and love God and love his neighbor as himself, thus to become virtuous. In the classroom, I exert power mostly by the use of my words, supplemented by grades and behavioral punishments, if necessary. But like God, the one thing I want the most for my students I am unable to effect by employing my power.

My institutional authority as a teacher allows me to employ power, but the one thing I want most to do with my power is for students to recognize my authority freely, absent the use of my power, my authority, that is, as someone who uses his power to dispose them to recognize and love and obey the authority of Truth. This "outcome" I cannot "manage" effectively because ultimately it is a free choice of each student. The most I can do is to point to this authority and try to make it attractive to them. The paradox here is that the more students recognize that this is my aim, the less effective my use of the strategies of classroom management is because they know that I can't coerce them to achieve this aim, which is really the aim that they have for themselves if they knew themselves the way I know them. Those students who recognize this and choose to make God and Truth their authority don't need classroom management strategies because they have become independently motivated for the right end and under the right authority, God, and so respecting my authority, which is ordered to His, and listening attentively and with docility to my words, mostly Socratic questions, and obeying the few, gentle "management" directives I give from time-to-time to help them achieve their good as students, that is, my employment of power, is something they genuinely want to do freely and without the need of any coercion.

On the other hand, those students who have not chosen to obey the higher authority that I miserably try to represent will find being on task and engaged difficult, as for them, I am just another power broker, which is dehumanizing to them. They are right to rebel against this. But as long as they are not preventing the other students from obtaining the good they have chosen to obtain, I can't do any more for them, and I need to allow them some leeway. This means that I must tolerate them being uninterested and sometimes a bit distracted and even distracting to others. If I were to exert coercive power to make sure that they were on task and engaged, for the sake of an "effectively managed classroom," it would hurt the common good of the class, for the classroom atmosphere would become bureaucratic, cold, and authoritarian (like those movies that show classrooms in China or in Ireland in the 50s with mean nuns with rulers), and the content would need to be essentially busy work with clear "objectives." I could easily exert the exact amount of coercive power to make these power-oriented students "behave," but this would hurt not only the more mature, authority-oriented students, but also them because what they need is to be (relatively) free to reject my authority, and deal with the natural and supernatural consequences of their rejection, not just my stupid punishments.

If the consequences of my power are the only consequence they experience of their rejection of true authority, such as scolding, detention, moving their seat, sending them out, getting a bad grade, then they might be inclined to think that power is all there is, and this may very well be the reason they are rejecting my authority in the first place, because perhaps in the past the authority figures they had to deal with were actually just power figures, and they rightfully rebelled against these loveless frauds. They are right to think of me as the same as these frauds and traitors, at least at first, and so I need to be patient with them and not use my power willy-nilly. After all, I was one of these students, and I only was able to recognize my foolishness by experiencing someone who loved me enough to use his authority and power to help me to realize what authority really is.

Consider Jesus the Teacher. What did He want? He wanted everyone to whom He spoke to recognize the authority of the Father, which was, of course, also His own authority, but they needed to see His own power-rejecting obedience to the Father to understand the difference between power and authority. Such was the sole purpose of His employment of power, sometimes miracles of healing, sometimes violence—overturning the temples and whipping people—sometimes just the heart-melting power of His loving words and actions. At a certain point, after His resurrection, He destroyed the Jewish Temple, but this was for the same purpose, to show the Jews that power wasn't authority. Most of them did not listen.

He didn't use "management techniques." "Philip saith to him: 'Lord, shew us the Father, and it is enough for us.' Jesus saith to him: 'Have I been so long a time with you; and have you not known me? Philip, he that seeth me seeth the Father also. How sayest thou, shew us the Father?'"[5] This was all Jesus could say and do, for He was literally powerless to "manage" their ability and decision to see the Father in Him. It is the same for all teachers. Teachers are powerless in the very thing they want the most, that students recognize in their teacher and their teacher's words as nothing but a pointer to Reality, to Authority, to the Father, and that they learn to see in all words and all events and all that they experience that same pointer. This is the essence and purpose of classical education.

Naomi Wolf tells us why she didn't go along with the demonization of the unvaccinated when all her leftist friends did, who were, by definition, against unjust discrimination.[6] She didn't go along with it because she could see that it was unjust, and one simply doesn't do or go along with injustice. Her friends, by doing and going along with injustice, revealed that they had never really been against injustice but only pretended to be so as to gain something from the world. Naomi lost these friends, who at this point saw her as an enemy, and since then she has been writing and speaking about the hypocrisy of the left as well as her awakening to the spiritual world, especially the reality of deep, supernatural evil. Her decision whether to stand against injustice, knowing it would mean the loss of her reputation, was a trial and judgment, and she passed it. Many of us went through a trial like hers, and many failed it. The plandemic was a judgment on the world, and it was allowed by God to be a preparation and foreshadowing of another and more momentous judgment that looks to be soon upon us.

---

[5] John 14:8-9, Douay-Rheims Bible.

[6] Naomi Wolf, *Facing the Beast: Courage, Faith, and Resistance in a New Dark Age* (White River Junction, VT: Chelsea Green Publishing, 2023).

Authentic prophecy, private revelation, the testimony of mystics, and Sacred Scripture and Tradition all point to a future event where every human being alive on earth at the same moment will experience a judgment of and on their soul. This event has been called The Warning and The Illumination of all Consciences.[7] It will be a day in which God will supernaturally illuminate the conscience of every man, woman, and child on earth. Each person would momentarily see the state of his soul through God's eyes and realize the truth of His existence. At this moment, there will only be authority, pure authority, authority alone, with no admixture of power, no coercion, no incentive, no reward or punishment, no social pressure, nothing but authority. And only one choice will be possible, either to obey or disobey this authority, with only two possible moral objects, either absolute good or absolute evil, and with only two possible intentions, to obey authority *because it is authority,* or to disobey authority because it is authority. It will be as if taken back in time to the foot of the cross to behold Jesus crucified, Authority in the flesh. Do you recognize it? Here is Truth Incarnate. The Truth. How do you respond? You will not now be able to consider consequences or benefits or reasons. No one is watching you. No power is talking to you. Here is just pure authority. The authority of truth on a cross as the authority of the truth about your soul. What will you do?

This moment will be just a supernatural focusing and heightening and intensification of what each moment of our lives truly is, though we tend not to see it. We are always in the presence of one

---

[7] https://afterthewarning.com/the-illumination/the-warning/the-coming-illumination/.

authority or another, although there is really only just one, for authority is the justification and basis for our every thought, word, and action, for all of our exertions and displays of power, whether we recognize it or not. My fingers are typing right now and are empowered to do so by an authority, the authority of my will. My will is empowering my fingers to type as commanded by the authority of my mind. And my mind and will are mutually empowered to command and act by the authority of the Good, or, at least, what my mind through its concepts and my will through its rational desires judges to be the Good, and, at the very moment of decision, what *I* judge to be the good action here and now in light of the ultimate Good that transcends the here and now, God.

The problem is that unlike at the future moment of Illumination where we will be alone and faced with True Authority—and nothing else—we are always confronted with competing authorities, or rather, one real authority beckoning our recognition and obedience, and a myriad of unreal seductive or menacing counterfeits. Neither of these can compel our recognition and obedience, for regardless of the coercion employed to manipulate us or the prospects of power promised to seduce us, we are always free to choose which authority we recognize and obey. But how is true authority to be recognized and how are the counterfeits to be unmasked and resisted?

I wish I could give a simple answer to this. Ultimately, answering this question correctly and acting upon it at every moment is one's salvation, so everyone needs to answer this question for themselves. But if you are not quite able to figure it out in time for the Warning, God will answer it for you then, for this is what the Warning really is, and this is why it is the culmination of God's unfathomable mercy. But in the meantime, let us try to answer it, at least in general terms, and we will use the plandemic to help us, for it was a dress rehearsal for the Warning. But first, read this amazing passage by the 20th-century theologian Karl Rahner:

There is an individual who discovers that he can forgive though he receives no reward for it, and silent forgiveness from the other side is taken as self-evident. There is one who tries to love God although no response of love seems to come from God's silent incomprehensibility, although no wave of emotive wonder any longer supports him, although he can no longer confuse himself and his life-force with God, although he thinks he will die from such a love, because it seems like death and absolute denial, because with such a love one appears to call into the void and the completely unheard of, because this love seems like a ghastly leap into groundless space, because everything seems untenable and apparently meaningless. There is the person who does his duty where it can apparently only be done, with the terrible feeling that he is denying himself and doing something ludicrous for which no one will thank him. There is a person who is really good to another person from whom no echo of understanding and thankfulness is heard in return, whose goodness is not even repaid by the feeling of having been selfless, noble, and so on. There is one who is silent although he could defend himself, although he unjustly treated, who keeps silence without feeling that his silence is his sovereign unimpeachability. There

is someone who obeys not because he must and would otherwise find it inconvenient to disobey, but purely on account
of that mysterious, silent, and incomprehensible thing that
we call God and the will of God. There is someone renounces
something without thanks or recognition, and even without
a feeling of inner satisfaction. There is a person who is absolutely lonely, who finds all the bright elements of life pale
shadows, for whom all trustworthy handholds take him into
the infinite distance, and who does not run away from this
loneliness but treats it with ultimate hope. There is someone
who discovers that his most acute concepts and most intellectually refined operations of the mind do not fit; that the
unity of consciousness and that of which one is conscious in
the destruction of all systems is now to found only in pain;
that he cannot resolve the immeasurable multitude of questions, and yet cannot keep to the clearly known content of
individual experience and to the sciences. There is one who
suddenly notices how the tiny trickle of his life wanders
through the wilderness of the banality of existence, apparently without aim and with the heartfelt fear of complete ex-
haustion. And yet he hopes, he knows not how, that this
trickle will find the infinite expanse of the ocean, even
though it may still be covered by the grey sands which seem
to extend forever before him. There is God and his liberating
grace. There we find what we Christians call the Spirit of
God.8

---

8 Karl Rahner, *The Practice of Faith: A Handbook of Contemporary Spirituality*, trans. David Morland (New York: Crossroad Publishing Company, 1986), 82-

What do these grace-filled words from Rahner tell us about authority?

Jesus told Luisa Picarretta:

"When Pilate asked Me whether I was King, and I answered: 'My Kingdom is not of this world, for if It were of this world, millions of legions of Angels would defend Me'. And Pilate, on seeing Me so poor, humiliated, despised, was surprised, and said with greater emphasis: 'What? You are a King?' And I, with firmness, answered him and all those who are in his position: 'I am King, and I have come into the world to teach the truth. And the truth is that it is not positions, nor kingdoms, nor dignities, nor the right of command that make man reign, that ennoble him, that raise him above all. On the contrary, these things are slaveries, miseries, which make him serve vile passions and unjust men, making him also commit many unjust acts which disennoble him, cast him into mud, and draw the hatred of his subordinates upon him. So, riches are slaveries, positions are swords, by which many are killed or wounded. True reigning is virtue, to be stripped of everything, to sacrifice oneself for all, to submit oneself to all. This is true reigning, which binds all, and makes one loved by all. Therefore, my Kingdom will have no end, while yours is near to perishing.' And, in my Will, I made these words reach the ear of all those who are in positions of authority, to let them know the great danger they are in, and to

---

83.

put on guard those who aspire to positions, to dignities, to command."[9]

What is the ultimate purpose of evil? What do demons and the most evil people want most for those to whom they do evil? They want their victims to obey power and not authority, for this is the definition of sin, and they want most of all for us to choose Hell over Heaven, preferably at every moment but especially at the moment of our death. What those vignettes articulated by Rahner display so beautifully and profoundly are examples of people choosing authority over power, the authority of what the existential moment in which they found themselves called for, of what the reality they were now experiencing dictated, of what God speaking to them right now in their unique and particular circumstances was asking from them. In every one of these examples, there was another choice available to them that would have brought them some increase in personal power or prestige, psychological well-being or emotional satisfaction, worldly stability or justice. Yet they did not choose it, and what they did choose brought them a decrease in these things without any apparent compensation. Why would they choose such a thing?

If I tried to answer by saying that they were aware of some other more obscure and spiritual good that they would obtain by renouncing the more worldly one, then these would no longer be examples of people choosing authority over power, just people choosing a less obviously worldly kind of power over authority. The true answer is that they chose authority over power because at this moment, God's will, not their own, was what they wanted most. "Not my will by

---

[9] Luisa Piccarreta, *The Book of Heaven*, vol. 15, July 5, 1923.

thine be done." And why they or anyone else chooses this is a mystery. What we do know is that unless we want this, unless we desire salvation over well-being and authority over power, we will not go to heaven after our death. In the choice they made at that moment, they defeated evil, and the demons and evil people who are now doing everything in their power to get us to choose hell can be defeated by no other way than for us to choose authority over power, salvation over well-being, God's will over our own will at every moment of our lives, and especially at the moment of our death. If it weren't for God having become a man and stripping Himself of everything, sacrificing Himself for all, and submitting Himself to all, we wouldn't know the true nature of and difference between authority and power, salvation and well-being, Heaven and Hell, and if it weren't for Him doing it on our behalf, we wouldn't be able to choose the one and reject the other.

In the Warning, God will reveal to us all the times that we didn't make the right choice, when we allowed evil to win and bring us closer to Hell. There will be no possibility of not seeing the truth about ourselves. He will just show it to us, and He will not threaten us with future punishments or attract us with future rewards. We will be in an analogous situation to the people described above right before they made their choices. We will be free to respond to what we see in the way we are always free to respond to each moment of our lives with a choice to obey authority or power. The difference is that at this moment, there will be no way of avoiding the truth that one has either chosen for authority or power, and one will completely and clearly understand what this means. There have been dress rehearsals for the Warning, such as the plandemic.

Evil people inflicted fear on you in 2020 to get you to choose power over authority, to choose power *as* authority. They wanted you to reject truth as your authority. Normally, one chooses truth because it doesn't cause much pain to do so, and the rewards are good ones. It's not clear that one is choosing truth for its own sake, though, because of the power accompanying it, such as the power to preserve one's life by accepting the natural truth of gravity, or the social power one achieves from obeying the moral truth that people generally like you when you are good to them, and they tend to be good to you back. You gave into this fear, and at some point, they lied to you about the masks and the lockdowns and the injection. In normal circumstances, you would have wondered if what was being told to you was the truth, since it was obvious that masks wouldn't protect you that much, if at all, from a very small virus, and if they cared about your life and it were as deadly as they said, why would they want you to risk death by going outside wearing a flimsy piece of cloth and walking only one way in supermarkets? Then they wanted to force you to get an injection, but you kind of knew it wasn't tested adequately. In any event, you knew it was wrong to believe things that very well could be untrue, and you would have asked questions to find out, but in this case, doing so meant a loss of power. You decided to choose to obey the authority of probable lies over justified truth because of the power it gave you, and thus you let evil get its way with you—and you took a step closer to Hell. But you were proud of your decision for Hell and you and your new friends bragged about it to each other and abused those who chose Heaven. And you told yourself that you were the ones who chose to love yourself and others and obey the truth and authority. No, you loved nothing and obeyed Satan.

If you haven't repented of this, you're not going to do well during the Warning. Why would you choose truth over lies when God shows it to you directly when you didn't choose it when He showed it to you indirectly through your own power of reason and the advice and admonitions of others you knew were trustworthy? Why would you choose authority and salvation over power and well-being now if you didn't then? It will be even harder for you now because you will get only pain from doing so and pleasure from rejecting it. This is your own doing. God will not coerce your decision, just as He didn't then. And if you choose against Him now, you may never have a chance to choose for Him ever again.

God allows demons and evil people to coerce us with fear or pleasure so that He can see what we will choose when choosing Him means choosing against what will rid us of the fear and being us pleasure. This is what the plandemic was all about, and it looks like most Catholics chose against Him, including most of the bishops and priests as well as the occupier of the See of Rome. God also brings us into the dark night of the soul when He thinks we are ready, during which He Himself afflicts us, out of love, for the same purposes of spiritual trial. Whether evil does it, permitted by God out of love and justice, or He does it, God is now putting before us a choice between authority and power, salvation or well-being, love or self, His will or our own, and He is trying to get us to see that the stakes for our choice are either Heaven or Hell. Don't wait until the Warning to make your choice. Repent, and choose God Alone— now.

And we beseech you, brethren, by the coming of our Lord Jesus Christ, and of our gathering together unto him. That you be not easily moved from your sense, nor be terrified, neither by spirit, nor by word, nor by epistle, as sent from us, as if the day of the Lord were at hand. Let no man deceive you by any means, for unless there come a revolt first, and the man of sin be revealed, the son of perdition, Who opposeth, and is lifted up above all that is called God, or that is worshipped, so that he sitteth in the temple of God, shewing himself as if he were God. Remember you not, that when I was yet with you, I told you these things? And now you know what withholdeth, that he may be revealed in his time. For the mystery of iniquity already worketh; only that he who now holdeth, do hold, until he be taken out of the way. And then that wicked one shall be revealed whom the Lord Jesus shall kill with the spirit of his mouth; and shall destroy with the brightness of his coming, him, Whose coming is according to the working of Satan, in all power, and signs, and lying wonders, And in all seduction of iniquity to them that perish; because they receive not the love of the truth, that they might be saved. Therefore God shall send them the operation of error, to believe lying: That all may be judged who have not believed the truth, but have consented to iniquity.[10]

Jesus Christ, the omnipotent, came to save us from enslavement to power. He did this by overpowering the powers of this world, not with His almighty power, but with his divine authority. When he

---

[10] 2 Thessalonians 2:1-12, *Douay-Rheims Bible*

told Pilate that He could at any moment summon legions of angels to defend Him, but would not do so due to His Kingdom being "not of this world," He was telling Pilate and us that authority trumps power, and the kingdom based upon true authority is sovereign over all others. The Jews rejected Him because they worshipped power, their own, and He both refused to join in their idolatry and unmasked it as such. The Jewish leaders crucified Authority itself, and any person from that day on who knowingly and deliberately rejects the divine authority of Jesus Christ does the same.

There were foreshadowings of Christ's unmasking of power without authority in both the Old Testament—consider Jeremiah's call to surrender and Isaiah's Suffering Servant—and in pagan literature, the *Iliad* being, as Simone Weil has shown, an unmasking of the collective suicidal delusion of the archaic worship of force, with the reconciliation between Achilleus and Priam hinting at the transcending of this worship. But it was the Passion of Our Lord, the ultimate epiphany of power with no authority in His murderers, and authority with no power in His crucified helplessness, that fully unmasked and conquered the satanic system of the sovereignty of power with no authority and authority annihilated by power. It would take a thousand years or so for the pagan-power system to be fully repressed (but certainly not destroyed, for both anti-Christian Judaism and paganism lived on underground, as it were) and the Christian system to be substantially incarnated in Western society. But as Andrew Willard Jones demonstrates, the deterioration and fragmentation of the Medieval system of universal peace over violent conflict and divine authority over demonic power in the fourteenth century within the metaphysical acid of nominalism led to

Protestantism, confessionalization, the "Wars of Religion," and the rise of the sovereign nation-state, in which spiritual power was made subservient to temporal power. Well before the manifestly diabolical French Revolution, the pagan power system was for all intents and purposes back, though now wielded by Christian sovereigns and peoples:

> After this period, the relationship between rulers and their subjects changed. Previously, people tended to have overlapping religious and political loyalties and associations. No one ruler could claim all of a person's obedience. Instead, societies tended to be diverse, with local authorities, such as the local lord and bishop, sharing most direct authority, and with these small groupings united into larger ones in similarly diverse ways. Any given person had a wide range of relationships with a wide range of authorities, including universal authorities, such as the emperor and the pope, that transcended all local power. Now, however, it was agreed that the people of each country were solely subject to a single state. This was not a division of religion from politics because nearly all the states of Europe were confessional states, with highly centralized churches, but it was the positioning of politics, of the temporal power, as the only real human power. The spiritual was entirely subservient to it and operated entirely within its bounds. Each country would decide what religion was and how it would function inside its own borders, and other countries were indifferent to its actions.

Wars between countries, then, would no longer be over spiritual things but over merely temporal things like natural resources, power, or eventually ideology.[11]

"The temporal power as the only real human power." This has been the case ever since, and it has only become more pronounced and institutionalized. Unless it is institutionally reversed, with power in complete submission to authority, no personal or private employment of power, however benevolent, graced, and aimed at the Good, will do the amount of good that is required and desired by God. And such a reversal now cannot be accomplished by the employment of merely human power, just as the original overthrow of the system by Jesus was not accomplished by power. It can only be accomplished by the omnipotence of authority, ultimately of truth, which is to say, by the authority of truth taking the place of power in both the souls of individuals and society at large.

The scamdemic was the global enthronement of power without authority and was permitted by God as a trial and test for Christians in preparation for the reign of Antichrist, a trial and test which they, as a whole, failed. By now, it is clear to many of those—but not enough!—who knew right at the beginning that the pandemic was based upon lies, a coordinated and orchestrated psy-op, that it was and is something even more evil than this, namely, an all-out war by the satanic elite against, literally, the whole world, to end in the death of billions and the complete physical and spiritual enslavement of the rest. But though the enemy employs massive and deadly physical

---

[11] Andrew Willard Jones, *The Two Cities: A History of Christian Politics* (Emmaus Road Publishing, 2021), 165.

terrorism as a tactic, its main goal, getting its marching orders from Lucifer himself, is the damnation of souls. Thus, its main weapons are not physical, but psychological and spiritual—intimidation and seduction. They are now winning this war, in my estimation, for the masses of the world have capitulated to its intimidation and seduction. This didn't have to happen, and it doesn't have to happen now or in the future. They can only win the war for our souls with our free cooperation.

Just as a temptation from the Devil has power over us only to the extent it is consented to, a lie has power only when it is believed, and the most power when it is deliberately preferred to the truth. And this is precisely what happened in March 2020. Those who should and could have known better surrendered to power with no authority, knowing, or at least suspecting, that it had no authority. How do we know this? Because, by and large, the claims they made were not questioned as to their truth, and the measures that were implemented were not questioned as to their goodness. And anyone who did question them was mercilessly attacked by these unquestioners and deemed to be evil. But to accept a claim that is neither self-evidently true, previously known to be true, nor made by a credible authority without questioning it in the light of truth is to sin against and betray the authority of truth. Moreover, these claims were used to justify the use of power, what was soon to be manifested as a tyrannical and totalitarian employment of power the likes of which had never been seen in human history. But to exert or condone the use of power without questioning its goodness, a power not seen to be justified by the authority of the Good, is also to sin against and betray the authority of Truth, the Truth about the Good.

We could have defeated the whole scamdemic and all the connected evil that has ensued in its wake up to the present time, as well as conquered the enemies of Truth who now rule us with an iron grip, by simply asking questions about their eminently questionable claims and unjustified exertions of power: Is it true, based upon what I can see with my eyes and what tradition has taught me and what I know from experience about health and sickness, that we are really in the midst of a deadly pandemic? Why was a sophisticated simulation of virtually the same Covid-19 pandemic scenario held in October of 2019? Why are the hospitals putting so many people on ventilators when this was never done before and is killing more people than it is saving? Is Ivermectin really just a horse dewormer? Do masks really protect us from viruses that are way smaller than the mask mesh? Are the CDC and the WHO and Anthony Fauci and my town's public health officer completely authorized to issue commands that trump all other authorities as well as settled law? Does the governor of my state have the right to shut down the economy without the consent of the people and that of state representatives? Does the Pope have the right to cancel Holy Week? Why are exceptionless and constitutionally protected rights suddenly abrogated by fiat, and at the behest of unelected, globalist bodies? Why is the sacred political principle of subsidiarity being violated on every level? Why are doctors and scientists who question anything certain public officials claim being censored and canceled? Why are questions being prohibited and the people who ask them treated like traitors and violent criminals?

A person asking questions regarding the claims and actions of those in power indicates that he holds the truth and the good to be ultimate authorities, not the claims and actions themselves or the people and groups who make and do them. But not only did most Christians not ask these questions, but they also mocked and persecuted those who did. If you would have asked these Christians if they believed they had personal access to the truth and the good, and the obligation and responsibility to ensure that everything they believed and every action they did or permitted to be done to them was acceptable only by the authority of the truth and the good, they would have assured you indeed they did believe such. But, as a whole, they showed only lip service to these beliefs in how they responded to an intimidating and seductive power demanding their allegiance and rewarding them for giving it. There were many, of course, due to prolonged conditioning in a culture of power worship and bereft of counteracting conditioning in sub-cultures of theistic belief and practice, who really did not believe in the authority of transcendent and absolute moral and spiritual truth and goodness, and these were sitting ducks for the totalitarian onslaught. They gave in immediately and with pleasure. But many did not explicitly or consciously believe in transcendent authority, who would have even mocked such authority as superstitious and unenlightened and oppressive, but who yet acted as if they did believe by asking truth-seeking questions to power and courageously resisting its commands—and suffering a lot for it. But the many well-formed Christians, particularly Christian leaders, had no excuse, and they committed treason against the sacred authorities they should have honored. Under the extreme duress and seduction purposely unleashed on us by the Satanists, it was difficult. But this is what it means to be a Christian. They showed their real colors—the colors of hypocrites, liars, and cowards. Some repented of their treason, but not nearly enough to make a difference. Christians lost this all-important spiritual battle, and we are not in good stead for the next one.

What the Scamdemic revealed was that the vast majority of religious believers in America were and are, underneath pious externals, either liars or cowards, for when the demand to offer the pinch of incense to the Satanic Caesar was made, they did it, showing their ultimate allegiance to Power over Authority, to Power without Authority. If all or even most of these repented, even now, I wouldn't be writing this article. But I have seen no sign of mass repentance. If anything, there is a doubling-down. They could have asked questions, and when their questions were not answered, they could have refused to believe unjustified claims and obey unjustified commands. They freely chose and are now still freely choosing not to. I daresay Christians still can defeat this ongoing totalitarian onslaught simply by disobeying power with no authority. If we had done this in 2020, the totalitarians would either be in jail right now or dead by execution for crimes against humanity.

The scamdemic and all that came in its wake, the Globohomo-trans cult, the Ukrainsane, and the CBDC program, as well as the emergence of an Antichurch fully on board with all these evils counterfeiting and attempting to replace the real Catholic Church, are all unprecedented crimes against humanity and God. But, they are only the precursor, the anti-John-the-Baptist to the Antichrist, as it were, preparing souls by a baptismal rite of mortal sin and the preaching of unrepentance for the final spiritual test and trial. Those who allowed themselves to be satanically baptized into power-worship and unrepentance will be judged, and their judgment will be their total enslavement to power without authority, the very definition of the Antichrist:

> Whose coming is according to the working of Satan, in all power, and signs, and lying wonders, And in all seduction of iniquity to them that perish; because they receive not the love of the truth, that they might be saved. Therefore God shall send them the operation of error, to believe lying: That all may be judged who have not believed the truth, but have consented to iniquity.[12]

Our mission now is to fight against the precursor of Antichrist with all our strength, but not with the worldly and illusory strength of power, but only with the infinite power of authority. How do we do this? Simply by ensuring that all we say and do, any word we speak, any employment of and obedience to power is aimed first and foremost at manifesting to ourselves and others the authority of the True and the Good, ultimately Jesus Christ and His Church. If we had all done this in 2020, the Luciferians' war against humanity would have been defeated before it began. It is not too late now to employ the power of authority for the salvation of humanity.

We must prepare ourselves spiritually for the arrival of Antichrist and help those who have received the love of truth, but who may not be quite prepared for this next and final test and trial. I fear that those who have not received the love of truth, who refused and still refuse to ask questions of power, may be lost. But we can still

---

[12] 2 Thessalonians 2:9-12, *King James Version*.

pray for them and must do so, for God's mercy is infinite and in-comprehensible.

There is No *Solution* to the Evil we Face

> I make evil problematical when I treat it as a kind of break-down that might happen in a piece of machinery, or as some-thing lacking, or as a functional failure. Evil reveals itself to me as, on the contrary, a mystery when I recognize that I cannot treat myself as something external to evil, as simply having to observe evil from the outside and map out its con-tours, but that on the contrary I am implicated in evil--just as one is implicated in crime. Evil is not only in front of my eyes, it is within me. . . .[13]

The great twentieth-century French Catholic philosopher, Ga-briel Marcel, wrote profoundly on the difference between a problem and a mystery. Here is a summary of his thought:

(1) A problem is an inquiry in respect to an object which the self apprehends in an exterior way without thinking of the self; a mystery is a question in which what is given cannot be regarded as detached from the self. I cannot define the question's answer without defining myself.

---

[13] Gabriel Marcel, *Man Against Mass Society*, trans. G. S. Fraser (South Bend, IN: St. Augustine's Press, 2008), 91.

(2) A problem admits of a solution, whereas a mystery can-
    not be solved for the questions ceaselessly renew them-
    selves, being unanswerable by any objective method.

(3) The impersonal knower can perform the experiment as
    if he were any trained observer in a problem, whereas in
    a mystery only the person as a person, that is, as a free
    being can choose how to respond to the question.

(4) Whereas in a problem the mind strives to master and
    control nature, in a mystery, the self is encompassed and
    mastered by a reality or experience greater than the self.
    without thinking of the self; a mystery is a question in
    which what is given cannot be regarded as detached
    from the self. I cannot define the question's answer
    without defining myself.

Aside from God, evil is the most profound mystery. And there
has never been as much evil in both the world and in the Church as
there is today. As modern Americans, a country, as Tocqueville told
us, was built by pragmatic problem solvers, we don't really know
how to deal with mystery. We want to turn all mysteries into problems, if we can even recognize a mystery, let alone behold it. This is
as true for Catholics as it is anyone else, though we should know
better, being that the religion we say we practice every day is nothing
but one, gigantic, unfathomable mystery. Canon law, Thomistic theology, and promulgated dogma do attempt to rationally articulate
and manage this mystery to some extent, but the distance between
the supernatural reality and these human mediations is still infinite,
though we often forget this. Contemporary managerial, therapeutic,

utilitarian, woke, capitalist culture sucks all the mystery out of life, and Catholic liturgy tends either to ape this aesthetic, as in the mainstream Novus Ordo milieus, or react against it mindlessly, as in Jansenistic and pharisee traditionalism. The return of the repressed in new age circles and the occult is less mystery than irrationality and demonic counterfeit. The mysterious is beyond reason, but it is not unreasonable. It is, in fact, the perfection of reason because it is the perfection of reality. God *is* mystery, and all created mysteries, such as the mystery of reason itself, of the human person, of his freedom, and of human love, participate in His uncreated mystery, which is the ground and fountain of all reality.

Both the mystery of God and the mystery of evil are revelations, so not realities that we can fully understand by our own intellectual powers. We may know *that* God and evil exist by our reason, but we can't know too much about them on our own. Catholics and other Bible-believing Christians are pretty good at recognizing and adopting the proper disposition toward the mystery of God in Himself, His unfathomable perfections and infinity; in His mysterious immanence in their personal lives and prayer, the mystery of His grace and mercy in their spiritual and moral lives; and the mystery of providence in human history, including His miraculous interventions in their personal histories. But though we experience evil, both in ourselves, in others, and in society at large, I'm not so sure that we are as good at recognizing it for what it is, for the incomprehensible mystery it is.

Right now, God is revealing evil in its purest form to us as it has never been revealed before, and if we are going to overcome and destroy it, which God wants us to cooperate with Him to do, we need to have the proper disposition towards it. Like God, it is first and foremost a mystery to be beheld, not a problem to be solved. One such mystery is the evil of the plandemic, as we have been discussing in this book, and particularly, the evil of those who planned it and who are planning the next one, and the evil of those who consented to their evil. The evil of those who planned it cannot be understood. The desire for money and power does not suffice. Bloodlust does not suffice. Psychopathy does not suffice. Ideology doesn't suffice. Demonic possession is an explanation, but how does one really explain that? Why would anyone want to be a slave to the Devil who hates you? These are all causal factors, of course. But those who planned the mass murder and total enslavement of the global population by the sorcery of portraying mass torture, domestic terrorism, and a deadly bioweapon as health protocols, with the ultimate goal of all of us voluntarily murdering our own bodies and souls, hate God, and they hate Him because He is God, not for any other reason. This is pure evil, and there is no explanation for it. None. It is because of this inexplicable, mysterious evil that God created Hell. Hell is a mystery that is also inexplicable, and those spiritual morons, such as David Bentley Hart, will have hell to pay for making Hell into a problem and then solving it by denying its existence. Oh, it exists, if only because those who planned the plandemic, such as Anthony Fauci and Bill Gates and Klaus Schwab, are already in it, indeed, are its incarnations, and only an eternity of punishment justifies their present and continued existence. Of course, they could repent, as our Faith tells us. That such is possible in their cases is a mystery I can't fathom.

It is also impossible to explain why billions of people consented to and defended the plandemic lies and crimes, after the time for invincible ignorance was over. This is also the mystery of evil. Ignorance doesn't suffice. Mass formation doesn't suffice. Fear doesn't suffice. Peer pressure doesn't suffice. These were all causal factors, but underneath and beyond them all is just surd evil, the unspeakable evil of betraying truth by either rejecting it outright or by not asking questions and searching for it. There is no explanation for this mystery. There is nothing more obvious to our souls that truth is the first and last authority for all our actions, and that it simply must be obeyed. That anyone would deliberately disobey the authority of truth is inexplicable. It is simply evil, and evil is a mystery. Hell must exist because of this evil. I am afraid that many will end up there because of their betrayal of the truth, calling good evil and evil good, which is the unforgivable sin against the Holy Spirit, unforgivable because unrepentable. One cannot repent and be forgiven if one rejects the authority of truth and identifies truth as lies and lies as truth, good as evil and evil as good. Again, all sins are repentable, even the "unforgivable" sin, but there is a good reason Jesus called it that. How can a sin be both forgivable and unforgivable? It's a mystery not a problem. Here's the proper response to it—Don't commit it. Millions did. Why? There is no explanation. It is a mystery. The mask is the sacramental of this unforgivable sin. The bioweapon injection is its sacrament.

We are witnessing the emergence of a group of bishops, priests, and laity who constitute the Body of the Devil hiding in the Church,

who are causing, not only by not restraining but also by actively promoting, the abominable evils unleashed after the inauguration of the
Great Scamdemic Lie:

—The now completely unrestrained spiritual and moral lawlessness and upside-down world of mutilation defined as loving
   affirmation and drag queens characterized as heroes and role
   models for children.
—The installation of the groundwork for genetically destroying
   most of the world's population with the rest living under
   complete mental and physical enslavement in Hunger
   Games silos euphemistically named "smart cities."
—Aggressive and mendacious military attacks based upon out-
   rageous lies and using gullible nations' young men as cannon
   fodder to trigger nuclear war at the behest of a global criminal mafia, all propagandized as "freedom and democracy."
   Add to all this evil the great apostasy embodied in the utterly
   diabolical "Synod on Synodality" that is set to be imposed by
   the antichurch on all the Faithful.

The Church must, before it is too late, name and condemn those
malicious personages and ruling groups of the unbaptized, including especially in elite positions of power, who reject both the Torah
and Jesus Christ and are imposing this rejection on the Christian
population. We need an all-out evangelization campaign, not useless
"dialogue." The Catholic prelates and laity who are traitors to the
Church must be unmasked and excommunicated. We must present
a strong, courageous, manly, authoritative Church, tempered by

genuine compassion and humility, to the world so that men of good will recognize in us their Lord. Our Lady of Fatima told us that the world would be chastised by the persecution of the Church, and I think we can see now what this means. The world needs to be rescued from itself by the Church, but the traitors within, as well as the cowardly, worldly, scandalous, and lukewarm, have rendered her all but unable to bear witness to the Truth and restrain the world's evil, let alone save it.

More evil is coming, and it is not a problem. If it were a problem, we could solve it. We can't. God, Who is mystery Himself, is the only one who can deal with the mystery of evil, and He has already done so. His name is Jesus Christ, Mystery Incarnate. But if we treat the evil we are experiencing as a problem, then we will prevent God from acting in and with us to defeat it, both in our souls and in the world. Such a defeat may require our martyrdom. We need intimacy with God to be able to receive such a gift. We need to live in His Divine Will.

Evil causes problems, and these we can attempt to solve. But the evil itself must be beheld, contemplated in the light of the mystery of Christ, and hated with all our heart, just as the mystery of God must be loved with all our heart. Perhaps if we hated evil enough, it would go away—or if not, we could defeat it by dealing with it head-on, as Christ did—but for this, we must love God enough, and we can only do that by admitting we can't, and begging His help every second of our lives. When we sin we hate Jesus without cause. That should make us stop. The Jews hated Jesus without cause. We know from Scripture that they will repent in the end. But now, and until then, we have the apocalypse, the unveiling, the fullness of the revelation of the mystery of evil. Pray for the conversion of the Jews. Surrender to the mystery of God by beholding Him on the cross, which was the mysterious revelation of both pure goodness and pure evil.

A Pandemic of Disobedience

God permits fallen angels and men to do evil for His greater glory, and so that He can bring more good to men and the world than would have been possible without it. God is like that. There is no exception to this truth, even when the evil is the unspeakable and incalculable and unfathomable evil of the plandemic. Does it get more evil than this?

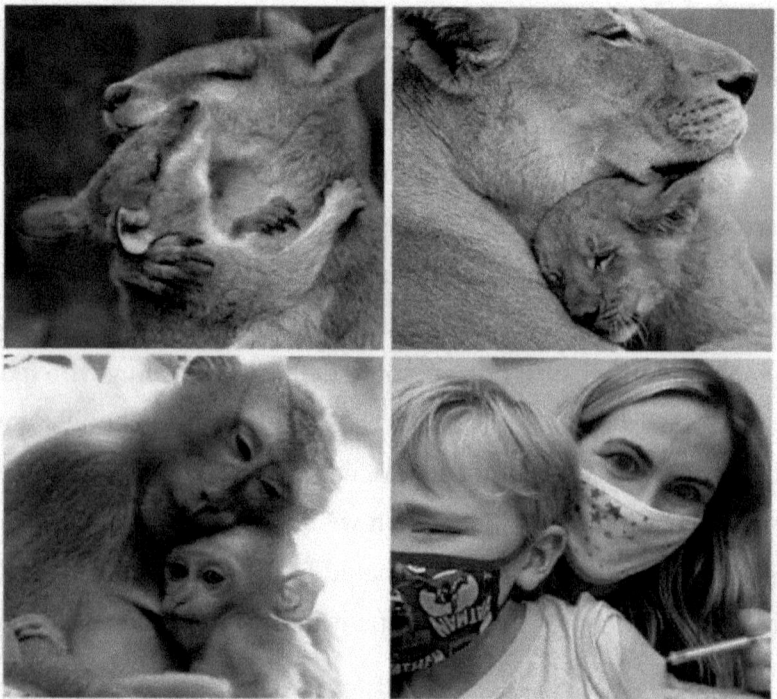

But what good could He bring to the world from His allowance of an elite of the demonically possessed, the psychopathic, the morally depraved, and the worshippers of Satan—some are all four—to commit the greatest crime against humanity in history, a global democide not just of bodies but of souls, aimed at manipulating every person on earth to commit the Unforgivable Sin? And, spiritually speaking, what could be worse than the visible leader of the Church founded by the Second Person of the Blessed Trinity promoting this satanic idolatry and mass formation as the epitome of Christian love, while mocking and denigrating those courageous and good souls who, obeying the Holy Spirit, won't bow down before this monstrous medical Moloch?

The truth is that there is nor can be nothing worse than this, except for what the future portends, absent divine intervention, which is the ever-increasing unfolding and metastasization of this unprecedented evil in scope, intensity, and depth. If this is correct, then the good that God plans to bring out of this evil, and is already beginning to do, must be the greatest good since the Incarnation, Death, Resurrection, and Ascension of the Second Person of the Blessed Trinity, which was itself preceded by the greatest evil ever committed by man, the deliberate murder of God. What could this second-greatest Good be, and how might it come about?

The murder of Jesus Christ, the first greatest evil, was the attempt to kill the God-man Himself, which succeeded—then failed. That failure brought about the greatest good, the descent of the Holy Spirit on earth and the institution of the Mystical Body of Christ on earth, for now the presence of God, which once existed only in the body and soul of a Jewish carpenter in Palestine, now living in

Heaven, could potentially inhabit the souls of all men, through Baptism, until the end of time. What brought about this new greatest good was the perfect obedience to God's will of one human being, Mary, and what brought about the greatest evil was the perfect disobedience to God's will of a group of people chosen from eternity and prepared specially by God to receive this gift. Of course, the evil was not exclusive to them, for as the Church has always maintained, all men in a mystical way were complicit in the murder of Jesus Christ, every time we commit sin.

And the same is true of the next-greatest evil in the history of humanity, the plandemic—we are all in some way responsible for it. Every act of cowardice, untruth, malice, idolatry, hypocrisy, betrayal—all have contributed to and caused the living hell we are undergoing. Some, of course, are more responsible than others, just as in the time of Jesus, and God will hold those in positions of authority and power, especially spiritual power, such as the Pope and the Bishops, much more accountable than the man in the street. But of all the sins that have led to the plandemic, one seems to me to be at the core of it, the sin of disobedience. And if this is true, then the plandemic will end through obedience, an obedience that will put an end to the Hell on earth we have incarnated and bring about the greatest possible good, the reign of God on earth as it is in heaven.

Those who planned the plandemic, I think, are beyond the reach of God's mercy, for they acted with a level of knowing malice that is damnable. If God chooses to grant them the grace of repentance, they are free to accept it, but honestly, I can't think of any scenario in which they would. When Jesus cried out to His Father from the cross, "Forgive them, Father, for they know not what they do," St.

Thomas Aquinas tells us that Jesus was *not* referring to the Pharisees and Sadducees who wanted Him crucified, for, as it is clear from the New Testament, they knew precisely what they were doing and whom they were crucifying.[14] It also seems to me that the great majority of media, academia, medical, pharmaceutical, tech, law, and government elites (particularly mask-loving board members of schools and public health officers of upper-middle-class cities) are probably in the same spiritual boat as the ultra-elite of the WEF, Big Pharma, WHO, CDC, NIH, FDA, Central Banks, etc. Their disobedience to God and the Tao seems quite knowingly malicious, and as the truth about the unspeakable crimes they have done, especially to children, becomes more clear, they only become more firm in their lies and malice and projection.

But the rest of us, either those who never bought into any of it; those who did, compromised with evil, but saw the light and repented; and those who from the beginning until now have obeyed the True and the Good, are still savable. For our disobedience was not out of diabolical malice, but fear or greed or mass formation psychosis, or perhaps just apathy, laziness, or stupidity. We are being called by God now to practice the supernatural virtue of obedience to a heroic degree, for we must repair and undo the countless infidelities and lies-to-self of others and ourselves that we have committed in the past, and we must attain to a new level of obedience to put an end to this nightmare once and for all. If we do so, God will give

---

[14] Thomas Aquinas, *Summa Theologiae*, III, Q. 47, Art. 6, Reply to Obj. 1, trans. Fathers of the English Dominican Province (New York: Benziger Brothers, 1947).

us literally heaven on earth, something He has been waiting to do for 2000 years.

Here's what the disobedience of the vast majority of human beings on the planet from 2020-2023 looked like: "I suspect that there is no law requiring masks, but I'll wear one because I am being told to do so, and I love obeying false authority, especially when so many others are doing it with me, because it means I don't have to obey the Truth that discomforts me. I suspect that viruses are too small for masks to work, which someone told me once, but I'll believe an expert who says otherwise anyway, because I will be considered a loving person by my fellow teachers. I suspect that my child will be harmed by wearing a mask, but I just don't want to homeschool her, so I'll go along with the narrative. I know that I am in charge of the schools in my area and my duty is to the good of families and children, but I have been given a lot of money to mandate masks and experimental injections, so I won't listen to any position that contradicts the goodness of masks. I need the money. I am pretty sure as a doctor that the vaccine isn't really a vaccine, and can probably do harm, but I need to keep my license, so I'll ignore what I know. I don't know if the vaccine is harmful or not, but I am not going to look at the evidence because Trump supporters might be the source of it, and I hate them and need to hate them for some reason. I like thinking that healthy people are sick because it feels good not to have to obey reality and to have other people join me in this disobedience, for I can then keep looking at the unreality of porn without feeling guilty. I like being a priest and telling people to wear masks because I hate telling them to stop sinning because it reminds me of my favorite sins that I do not repent of, and so this satisfies my need to feel like I am a good person and priest. I like being a bishop and telling people that wearing a mask and getting the vaccine is loving one's neighbor because I love to spite the real men I have met who actually love their wives, children, and neighbors, and it is just so satisfying to me in my narcissistic lovelessness to tear down real men. I know I am supposed to be responsible for my own health, but it's too scary for me and takes too much effort, so I just love believing that vaccines are all I need, not because I really think it's true, but because I can sort of get away with thinking it's true. I want to think that I am a good person more than anything, and wearing a mask and getting the vaccine makes me look and feel like a good person, and I want this more than I want the Truth about these things as well as myself, and I can easily exclude any information that suggests I am not a good person for doing these things by canceling, mocking, and scapegoating "them." I know I am supposed to uphold my oath to the constitution and protect the citizens of my county, but no other sheriff is doing this and I can easily get away with just towing the party line and this will be over soon anyway so I need to just do what I'm doing even though somethings telling me I'm betraying my office and letting evil occur. But I won't think about that right now."

But there is also the disobediences of the more righteous among us. Have we done everything we can do to resist, to know God, to love, to go against our own wills, to be heroically courageous, to get out of our comfort zones, to put aside those addictions and desires and slothful distractions that keep us from doing God's will at every moment? We who know and understand the evil and the good are called to a higher level of virtue and holiness. Let us pray to God for the courage and love to become embodiments of truth and reality for others.

2020 was a pandemic of disobedience to reality, to what one knows or suspects to be true and good, to love, to God. And God is allowing it "so that the hearts of many will be revealed" both to others and to ourselves. Before the plandemic, our "little" disobediences to our consciences, to what we knew was true and good, our willing small hypocrisies and self-serving "white" lies, our putting prestige and image over the reality of things, our virtue-signaling and sundry idolatries of pleasure, comfort, opinion, image—all of these didn't seem to amount to much, didn't really hurt anyone. But in 2020, it was revealed that these were causing children, even our own children, to be tortured and murdered, and on a mass scale. Because of our disobedience, we literally injected ourselves with the blood of murdered babies. We were joyfully enslaving ourselves, with no possibility of liberation, to malicious sadists. We were so in love with disobeying reality that we would rather have hell on Earth than His gentle rule, "My yoke is easy and my burden is light." Well, that's what we got, and will continue to get.

God in His mercy is allowing us to see the true upshot of our little disobediences, each of which pounds the hammer onto the nails of the cross, and this is why He is allowing Hell to come to us before we die and live in it eternally, so that we will finally realize what we are doing before it is too late. In the movie *Signs*, the protagonist, Preacher Graham Hess, loses his faith in God after his wife dies in a brutal car accident. Aliens then take over the earth and threaten to destroy it. Nothing can stop it but Hess repenting of his sin. Yes, one man's sin of infidelity to God would have caused the whole world to be destroyed. "When a man lies, he murders some part of the world." The plandemic was the global alien onslaught, and it was our little disobediences to Reality and God that caused it. It is His mercy that allowed this, so that it doesn't have to become His justice. And if we obey, He will give us the greatest good. What does obedience look like and entail? Nothing very special or magnificent or showy. In fact, it is simply to live the life of failure, in the world's eyes, which is triumph in God's eyes. The key to this is the Beatitudes:

> Often, people are wont to refer to someone as "blessed" to highlight a condition of acquired happiness: "Blessed is he that ...", "Blessed are you that ...". The beatitudes that we are used to, however, are very different from those proposed by Jesus! We say blessed are the rich, because their future is guaranteed, blessed is he who laughs because he does not know suffering, blessed is the violent person because he is powerful and does what he wants, blessed are the clever and the unjust because they know the way to success, blessed is the lustful because he is free and fully enjoys the pleasures of life, blessed is the vengeful person because he obtains honor, blessed are the persecutors because they will gain the favor of the powerful and earn rewards, etc. The consciousness of worldly blessedness is based on envy: lucky him, because he has what I don't. But Jesus completely turns this way of life upside down. He not only asks us to climb the mountain on a weekday, to struggle in order to meet Him in such an unusual place, to sit on stone, to appear as frivolous, annoying

and romantic idealists in the mood for a one-of-a-kind vacation, but affirms that true blessedness belongs to those who are poor, suffering, meek, chaste, thirsting for justice, merciful, peacemakers, and persecuted! All people who are failures. Those who today are considered as failures are those that Jesus calls blessed or to which He paves the way to blessedness. He asks us to recognize ourselves as failures, to be such ... This is too much! It is certainly a message beyond reason. Our society (which aside from what we might think we like as it is, otherwise it would be different) does not propose the Beatitudes of the Gospel to the destitute or the defeated, but offers three possibilities: to become bad and get away with illegal means, to destroy one's true identity by tirelessly searching for therapies to come up with one that works, ready for any compromise with one's own conscience, or to remain excluded and die in darkness. Jesus teaches that in the condition of being last a person can find the first treasure – acknowledging one's own nothingness, a blessed state. And so, blessed are the poor in spirit who know and live this condition by renouncing self-love, blessed are those who mourn and who know pain and deprivation, blessed are the meek who respond to the abuser or to offenses with patience and long-suffering, blessed are the merciful who do not take revenge but become the object of wickedness, blessed are the pure in heart for they consider the other as an end and never a means causing scandal, blessed are the peacemakers who live in defeat and whose voice is

never heard, blessed are the those who thirst for justice enduring injustice without committing any, blessed are the
persecuted for justice's sake and in the name of Christ, who
are the stones rejected by the world and the cornerstones.[15]

How to live the Beatitudes? Pray to God as much as possible and
look inside your soul and listen to His voice and obey what He calls
you to do at every moment according to your state of life and vocation. And always search for and love the truth. It's not rocket science.
In the *Republic*, Plato said that justice was "minding your own business." I can't put it better. One indispensable tool for knowing God
and what he wants us to do, which is to live in His will, is silence.
Spend twenty to thirty minutes, twice a day, reciting lovingly "Jesu-
Abba" in your mind, and when your mind gets distracted come back
to these words:

Now you wish to empty yourself of all thoughts so that you
can be filled with the formless presence of God - Father, Son
and Spirit- the living Trinity that dwells within you. As you
continue in a relaxed manner to breathe deeply in and out,
synchronize your breathing with these two names who are
unseen but very really present: Jesus ... Abba. Breathe in
deeply and mentally recite the name and experience the presence of JESUS. Breathe out slowly and mentally say the name
and experience the presence of ABBA. Continue to breathe
in slowly and mentally think of Jesus. Breathe out slowly and

---

[15] Alessandro De Benedittis, "The Beatitudes," *Luisa Piccarreta: Official Web-
site, https://en.luisapiccarretaofficial.org/news/the-beatitudes/222.*

mentally think: Abba. Jesus ... Abba ... Do not be concerned about any thought content. Let the words become for you a way to rivet your attention and focus your mind so that you can reach a meta-rational state of concentration that will allow you to listen in a deeply receptive mood to God as He speaks to you in the utter silence of your body, soul and spirit. This is what it means to pray in the heart and in the spirit. It is to allow yourself to be filled like an empty receptacle with the Spirit's gifts of faith, hope and love. I believe this is what St. Paul was referring to when he told us that our recited prayers are not the highest form of adoration but that it is when we yield to the Spirit of Jesus and allow Him to pray within us that we pray the best.[16]

---

[16] George A. Maloney, *The Silence of Surrendering Love* (Notre Dame, IN: Ave Maria Press, 1976), 180.

Chapter IV

Apocalypse

From Apocalypse to the End of the World

Christopher Loughman: If it's all right, Dr. Kozinski, I'd like to quote from the introduction of your book for the sake of anyone unfamiliar with it:

> To its devotees, modernity is just the way things really are.... But to those more resistant and skeptical of its soteriology, modernity is Christendom's rotting corpse, having been murdered sometime in the Enlightenment by the sword of de-hellenization, the poison of nominalization and the stranglehold of secularization. And modernity has divided up the body, giving us Christ without the cross, in its liberal-democratic half, and the cross without Christ, in its totalitarian half. Modernity is nothing more than a counterfeit of and parasite on the Mystical Body of Christ.

Can we try teasing some of that out?

Thaddeus Kozinski: I think I would still agree with most of that. What we are dealing with now I don't think I could have imagined back then—the emergent global totalitarianism.

What I mean by modernity is more the ideology that accompanies public discourse and the way institutions function—the kind of implicit presuppositions and absolutes and the cult, the religious background that is inherent in modern life. What I am trying to do is reject the idea that [modernity] is just a kind of neutral space where one can freely live any type of life one wants without influence or conditioning or restrictions. I see it more as a kind of mood or background—the "imaginary," to use Charles Taylor's language—that has hidden metaphysical, theological, anthropological dogmas and customs and beliefs. So we need to be very wary and vigilant in order to detect them.

CL: Can we talk about how this applies to America? In section V of your book, entitled "Apocalypse," you speculate:

> Perhaps Lucifer employed his unimaginably powerful intellect to create and then immerse himself in an abstract and unreal universe of words—'liberty' and 'equality' come to mind—thereby severing himself from the concrete and real being of God.

Now I'm reminded that when Alexis de Tocqueville made his monumental survey of our young country in 1835, these were the two ideas he saw playing out in conflict here: the two you mentioned. "equality" and "liberty." And that conflict looked to him something like a closed dialectic, it looked to him something like the whole ballgame. We see these two ideas roughly manifest today in the camps of conservatism and small-l liberalism and that battle looks to many as if it's the whole ballgame. It's just the way things are.

One of the things you seem to be saying is that this conflict is not only not the whole ballgame, but that it's a counterfeit conflict delineating a counterfeit reality—and quite possibly something worse. Is that fair?

TK: My main foe is ideology—in the [Eric] Voegelinian sense of it as a kind of gnosticism, a kind of second reality. And what I am referring to about Lucifer is the ability of human beings to reject reality by repairing to abstractions and living life according to unreal universals. And when that gets institutionalized and enculturated, you wind up with an ideological culture. Add to this the technology and the complex institutions we have, the bureaucratization that takes us away from the ordinary activities of life, [you wind up with] the imposition of a counterfeit.

[This] counterfeit begins in the minds of philosophes and ends up for the masses being indistinguishable from the real. [As for] "liberty" and "equality," you have opposite sides of the spectrum using those terms, believing and behaving in the most dramatically antithetical manner. Ideology serves the oligarchs, not the public.

CL: In the same section of the book, you quote David Schindler: "The state cannot avoid affirming, in the matter of religion, a priority of either `freedom from' or `freedom for'—and both of these imply a theology." You then go on to say: "By prescinding from the particularity of religious truth in the organization of the American body politic, the American founders enshrined a theology, a religion. [And that] this religion's first commandment is the first amendment—and it does nothing less than separate the order of nature from the order of grace, person from faith and, indeed, freedom from truth itself."

Why do you think it was necessary to the founders that these profound separations occurred? What was the point?

TK: I don't want to condemn the American Founding simply because of what's come after it: the consequences of certain decisions they made out of circumstantial prudence based on the complexities of geopolitics, etc. It's extremely complicated, obviously. But if you look at something like the First Amendment:

To set up a constitutional regime and prescind from the order of religion, the supernatural, the reality of the Catholic Church....

It's the first time in history that a political order was set up where the cult, the sacred, the transcendent, the relationship to the divine is put wholly *within* the political order and, in effect, privatized: you have a first attempt at an a-religious political order.

CL: Is it as simple as Madison pitting our privatized belief systems against each other so that, for instance, the Catholic Church cannot establish hegemony?

TK: A lot of the Founders were hostile to the Catholic Church. John Locke, in the *Second Treatise of Government*, forbade two types of people from being good citizens in the new kind of commercial republic: the atheists and the Catholics. And that's because he knew that, for a Roman Catholic, political allegiance and citizenship were bound up with one's religious identity and the authority of the Church. Locke wanted the state to define what religion is and its place in the city. The state was going to limit itself and everything outside it. Whereas in Catholic political theology, it's not the state's prerogative to define the boundaries of church and state, of the sec-ular and the sacred.... It can't do it. [The state] can only do it if it already has an ecclesiology—in this case a Protestantized and deistic one. Locke says: "Every church is orthodox to itself." Meaning that no church has a from-the-inside monopoly on what's true in reli-gion. That statement itself denies the reality and authority of the Catholic Church.

And so, if you have a kind of political order that's based on this universal statement that there is no access to God's will that is an any way objective and authoritative for the public.... [No,] it's all a private matter. You can see the logic. What that implies. And what's going to happen.

CL: I hate to tell you how old I was when I learned that there was something very specific called "Americanism" and it was con-demned as a heresy by no less than Pope Leo XIII....

TK: *Testem Benevolentiae*, yes.

CL: And I don't think I'm unique in my ignorance. Now I had a terrific elementary Catholic school education, taught by bright, pi-ous, committed nuns.... But the pledge-of-allegiance, you know, was said with our morning prayers. And up on the wall behind the good sister, on each side of the crucifix, were pictures of George Washington and Abraham Lincoln and probably one of our first Catholic president Kennedy....

So that was the "social imagining," to use Charles Taylor's phrase, that we were immersed in. It all came at one as of-a-piece.

So, you know, being an American Catholic is...interesting.

TK: I had a similar awakening shortly after I was married. I was at a conference with Professor John Rao and the Dietrich von Hildebrand's group [The Roman Forum] at Lake Garda and I heard some talks given on Leo XIII and John Locke.

Before then, I was on my way to becoming a good neoconservative, going to Lord Acton conferences and the Heritage Foundation and the Philadelphia Society and all these things....

I had never read Leo XIII. Or if I had, I'd only heard about his economic encyclicals. I didn't know he had written about the Christian constitution of states or on Americanism or on freedom: *Immortale Dei, Testem Benevolentiae, Longinqua*.... The letter to the U.S. bishops where he says the Church has borne good fruit in America simply because it had a certain amount of physical freedom to do its work. But, he says, the Church would be better off of it wasn't dissevered and divorced, as it is in America, from the state.

A statement like that, from the pope, of course, got me thinking: What are the alternatives here? I thought theocracy was the kind of outdated, restrictive, repressive sort of state that we'd grown out of. But he's not talking about theocracy. And he's not talking about integralism, either.

D.C. Schindler does a great job with integralism: the solution is not to use the centralized, bureaucratic, Lockean state and import into it Catholic principles. The solution has to be much more radical and imaginative and therefore much different.

We see the problem as a kind of religion of Liberalism. D.C. Schindler has an essay called "What is Liberalism" in *New Polity*, and a book called *The Politics of the Real*, which I think is the best thing written on this topic. [He makes the compelling case] that if you want to know what modernity is, what liberalism is, [you have to ask]: What is it rejecting, most of all?

[The answer is] the Catholic Church. Not "Christianity." Not Christian "values," Christian principles. [It's rejecting] the *reality* of the Catholic Church. What-it-actually-is.

CL: And does this correspond to [D.C. Schindler's] explication of the [Lockean] inversion of the [Aristo-Thomist categories] of potentiality over actuality?

TK: Yes. That's in his first book of the trilogy he's writing, the first book [being] *Freedom from Reality*—that tremendous work on John Locke.

Because what that actuality is—the Catholic actuality—is the tradition that synthesized, once and for all, the Greek, the Roman, the Hebrew, the Germanic—all the tributaries of the axial age that came together with Christ. [The Incarnation] synthesized them all into a living reality, a lived tradition.

And what the Enlightenment represents in liberalism is [an attempt] to access these ingredients—the Greek sense of the truth and science, the Roman sense of the law and authority, the Jewish understanding of God's omnipotence and [man's] sin.... In Christ all of this is gathered up together. {And liberalism's approach winds up with] Humpty Dumpty. You can't separate them out. Once you try to access [these components] outside the Church's tradition they wind up becoming heresies. They end up becoming mad.

[And so] liberalism says: the Church and the tradition it embodies—not just intellectually, but morally, politically, in its economics and sociology, its [complete] living reality.... Liberalism says that it is not going to recognize this reality in our political order, in our laws and what we consider to be the human good.... [In its] rejection of reality it has to try to build upon something else.

Schindler says that liberalism has substituted the God of the Catholic Church, the true God, with "nature and nature's god." Well, what nature is this? What's this nature's god? It's a "potential religion"—it's pure potency overcoming actuality—which is impossible. There's no actual reality to it.

CL: Is that potency, that prioritization of potentiality.... Are we just talking about pure power at that point?

TK: Yeah, I think so. What makes you say that?

CL: Well, because ontologically [having bracketed the actual]—that's what you're left with. I think that's why we're steeped in power politics. Because that's all that's left.

TK: Yeah. And it's masked very well.

CL: It certainly is.

TK: Well, it's becoming unmasked now. My recent articles on Substack deal with what was implicit in early classical liberalism, [that it's manifesting now] as this monstrous, arbitrary power, a most inhumane diabolical dynamic. People are waking up to it because of the obviousness of it. And what they are doing is basically fighting it with old-school assertions of the Tao and simple goodness, the goodness of mothers and the working man in the street.

People without much higher education are seeing the basic realities. Because of the great evil we are undergoing they are recognizing the value of a human person and their ability to make their own decisions and to be cared for. When you're deprived of normal face-to-face conversations and you're in constant terror—propagandized—people are starting to realize: this is unreality. They may not put it that way. But they are actually demanding that the political order recognize the authority of reality.

When Schindler, for instance, says that liberalism is against reality, that it's potentiality over actuality, that liberalism is an all-out assault against the reality of the Catholic Church—what does that look like? Well, it looks like what we have today. It looks like the face of Fauci as savior.

CL: "Catholic" Fauci.

TK: [Laughs] You have someone telling us what to do in our public and private lives who has engaged in experiments putting monkey's heads in a tank to be eaten by sandflies or whatever it is….And he has experimented on human beings in the past, killing many and getting away with it. It's all in Robert F. Kennedy, Jr's recent book *The Real Anthony* Fauci. He is a psychopathic sadist, but he's our avuncular wise and loving man to whom we have given dictatorial authority over reality.

CL: You brought up the historian Dr. John Rao. And he said in a recent interview that in a time that loudly proclaims the separation of church and state as a given, that in fact there has never been greater unity of church and state but that it's an ironic if not inverted unity. And you recently quoted the theologian Chad Pecknold: "The progressive civic-religious regime is a very dangerous sort of pseudo-integralism, which is to say, an inverted parody of Christianity."

Now if this is true, then we are really through the looking glass.

Do you think it's just a matter of having a seat at the World Economic Forum and that the truth really doesn't matter?

TK: Yeah, that's a pretty low level of consciousness. I can't imagine a lower level of consciousness, actually, because what it comes down to, as we were saying, is pure power.

Being a person of faith means that you are not governed by pure power. You are governed by truth and love.

CL: You make the distinction between authority and power. I would think, given his transcendent concerns, he would be more committed to authority than he would be to pure power.

TK: Authority being reality.

CL: Right.

TK: Schindler says that authority is essentially generosity. That's what authority does—it gives itself, it gives reality, so to speak, so that power can do good work.

To call a literal poison good and to mandate it for children…. And for those people who [refuse to wear] the satanic sacramental of submission to arbitrary power—the mask—which everyone knows is medically useless and harmful—I think all this is the elites mocking us, like a diabolical liturgy.

I could use words like "diabolical disorientation" like Lucia at Fatima, we could talk about the antichrist and the spirit of antichrist, the great delusion, the prophecies of La Sallette and of other mystics…. But when you are actually living through it, it's literally incomprehensible.

CL: Something you maybe thought you would never see in your lifetime—the diabolical disorientation….

TK: But the thing that has shocked me most of all—and it's why we know we're in a kind of great tribulation—is the absolute complicity and cowardice of the clergy in shutting down the churches, in refusing to give the sacraments, and having their churches become "vaccine" sites—This is unimaginable stuff.

CL: You just mentioned scapegoating and one of my questions has to do with your interest in Rene Girard....

One of the more pernicious counterfeits going involves the therapeutic state and the grievance industry and it centers on the cult of victimization.

In the canon of the mass I attend, the priest references: "...a victim which is pure, a victim which is holy, a victim which is stainless...."

Now I have an impossible time—and mere cognitive dissonance doesn't begin to capture it—reconciling our Lord Jesus Christ with the mass media victim of various sexual and racial stripe that we are saturated with.

I think you go so far as to identify this manufactured victim as the new dominant oppressor. Of the new scapegoat.

TK: Girard makes a good case that the dynamic of scapegoating is the ultimate counterfeit salvation. The feeling you get from scapegoating another is instant self-righteousness in identifying all that is evil in the accused. You feel this sense of salvation and purification and you achieve [a type of] solidarity with your fellow scapegoaters. So, you have an enemy that you can project upon.

Girard shows that either you are allowing yourself to be the scapegoat—because you *are* guilty—but knowing that your Redeemer lives and has been scapegoated before you and therefore you will not be doomed and that the scapegoaters will not have the last word. The scapegoaters didn't write the Gospels.

Or *you* are going to be doing the scapegoating. There is no neutrality here.

And so what do we have with our culture right now? It's obvious that it's based on self-righteousness of the most cowardly, idolatrous and hypocritical people—the Covid-cult, the Covidians.... They are scapegoating those who will not accept this self-justifying community of the irrational—[clearly] totalitarian.

Now, the Church is supposed to be the one institution that doesn't do this. Every other institution will fall to it. [And so] it is not only doing it in its most elevated power structures—it's taking a lead in it.

I don't think Girard ever witnessed such a thing. He talks about certain things in the Middle Ages, when the Church got caught up in a kind of regression: pogroms, torture, etc. But if Girard were alive today, I don't know how he would understand what is happening.

CL: Your writing is not without some profound approaches to something like solutions. In a recent Substack article entitled: "The Only Way to Survive and Defeat the Satanic Plandemic," you quote Romano Guardini from The End of the Modern World:"

"The new age will declare that the secularized facets of Christianity are sentimentalities." And: "That the free union of the human person with the Absolute through unconditional freedom will enable the faithful to stand firm—God-centered—even though placeless and unprotected."

And while I hope everyone understands the controversies surrounding Karl Rahner, you forward this arresting quote from him: "The Christian of the future will be a mystic, or he will not be at all."

Now, we utilitarian Americans are built for something like the opposite of mysticism. So where does a typical American, specifically an American Catholic, begin?

TK: Well, the Catholics don't have a home anymore in most churches—the ones who are not Covidians are already being uprooted. But I have found a place with people I would never have dreamed I would be relating to in the last two years: new agers, atheists, animal rights people. [Laughs.] People who would normally be on the left, progressivists who have woken up, who feel alone and isolated. And we've come together in little activist groups against the mass insanity. People who are trying to love in the middle of this lovelessness. It sounds pretty hippie-ish, but it isn't. People have been brought to this position of needing each other. I see Guardini's prophecy coming true in ways I never would have thought when I quoted him.

In terms of mysticism.... To me [it means] being connected to what's real.... Whatever is the opposite of being a Covidian. [Laughter.]

But it's the life of prayer, mortification, the cross. I think it is also recognizing with Guardini that God is taking away the normal supports. We're talking about the possibility of being rounded up into concentration camps, of starving, of new diseases coming down the pipe. So if we are not crying out to God and asking to be in His will, mystically, so that we can know what to do and how to survive.... God wants us to call out to Him when we have nothing left. And I can't understand what is happening, the gravity of the evil—genocide, totalitarianism—I can't understand it unless I think of it as God saying: "Look, I'm letting this happen because I want you to depend on me completely. And I want to show you what happens when you don't." And that means that there is no more time, no more excuses—that when you pray, it has to be mystical. And mystical, to me, means complete surrender: be quiet, listen to God [in] the direct experience of God. As much as possible. Because we need it.

CL: It's not the Rod Dreher approach, "The Benedict Option?" I think you said somewhere that that's not even possible right now.

TK: No, that's not going to happen. Of course we have to flee from this cult and, as much as possible, the institutions that have enshrined it. We have to be present to each other, those who understand what is happening.

CL: Didn't Guardini say that at the end of the modern world the faithful are going to be lonely but that they'll find each other....

TK: Yes.

CL: ...but that it was going to be a lonely trek. It's not a sentimental view of what a Catholic is going to be looking at the end of the modern world.

TK: No. Another prophecy I want to bring up is by St. Louis de Montfort. In *The True Devotion to Mary* he says that saints in the end times will be the greatest saints in the history of the Church. And their greatness will be in their heroism and love and surrender. And Guardini says that the loneliness will be harsh, but the love will be greater. And so we'll be able to handle it.

And I wanted to bring up Luisa Piccarreta from Italy. I've been reading through her 36 volumes over the last few years. And from what I understand, she lived a life of virtue and holiness that was unprecedented, achieving for the world and the Church a new out-pouring of grace greater than all the others. It's called "The Gift of Living in the Divine Will." And when I read her writings and I try to understand what is going on right now.... It only makes sense that we need to be fused with Jesus Christ, to be one with Him in a way that is even higher than spiritual marriage.

It's not that anybody deserves this grace or that you can do it with your efforts. It's pure gift. It is being given to the world now and it's available to everyone.

So it's a new normal! And the new normal for Christians now has to be at this next level. Because what's coming down the pike.... I think we're just at the beginning. I don't like to say this. I say this with fear and trembling.

But I think there are also good signs. I don't keep my earthly hopes *up*—I keep them medium, as my son says. But there are some good signs that this two-year cycle is waning down and I don't know what's coming next. We need to keep on our toes and make God the priority.

Founding A Real Christian University in An Age Of Unreality

The Age of Unreality

Two decades ago, much talk existed globally of a "post-911" world and its permanency: "We're never going back to the world that existed before the Two Towers fell," we were told. Sometime in 2020, "The New Normal" was declared. Both these announcements signify paradigm shifts in global culture and mass psychology. Such shifts have occurred before in history, and we have learned all about them in our history books: From the Homeric to the Axial Age to the Dark Ages, from Medieval Christendom to the Renaissance and the Reformation, from the Enlightenment to the Industrial Revolution and to the Information Age. Is there anything unique or exceptional about this latest shift into "new normality," or is it just one more in a long litany of human cultural evolutions?

In 2020, all public Masses throughout the Catholic world during Holy Week were canceled. This has never happened—never—in the history of Christendom. The reason for the cancellation was, we were told, the worst plague in history. The fact that the Church was shut down—indeed, shut herself down—during her most sacred and otherwise inviolable celebrations reveals that this is a unique and exceptional paradigm shift. The paradigm shift that has occurred and is still underway, with each day witnessing an ever-deepening shifting, is, I maintain, a shift to the Age of Unreality. The most compelling evidence for the accuracy of this description is the fact that the Church herself has not only succumbed to this propaganda-concocted unreality, but has also taken a leading role in spreading it to the world.

As all the actual scientific evidence now indicates—and the data was available soon after March 2020 for those with eyes to see it and some conversance with credible alternative media journalism—no "pandemic" (in the traditional sense of the word, i.e., hundreds of millions of terminally sick and dead people all around the world) had actually existed. What existed was a treatable, mostly non-lethal disease with an infectious fatality rate comparable to the common flu. But there was a mass-casualty event, the mass deaths and injuries of those injected by a bioweapon masking as a vaccine. Yet, an official Vatican conference was held in May of 2021 that supported with spurious and tendentious moral and theological rhetoric the entire false narrative, its attendant propaganda, and its final cause and *raison d'etre*: the injection of the entire global population with what the consensus of true science indicates is, not a vaccine at all, but an experimental, untested, and manifestly harmful—and fatal for a significant number—gene-altering serum.

As the abovementioned facts indicate, we are truly in uncharted waters: a worldwide propaganda onslaught the scale and malice of which the world has never seen hypnotizing the global populace into state of psychotic fear in which millions consented to, or at least did not widely and forcefully resist, a global economic shutdown—a crime against humanity on a massive scale. This shutdown included a deprivation of fundamental human rights, the physically and psychologically dangerous and medically useless masking of whole populations, including young children, and the coercive program of injecting every living human being with a untested, gene-altering serum, all for a disease that according to the actual numbers is no more fatal than the flu. Add to this the official endorsement of this totalitarian program by vast majority of Catholic clergy—indicated by closing of Churches, refusing to hear confessions or give Last Rites, mandating masks and social distancing, and even using their parishes as injection sites (not to mention the ever increasing celebration and normalization of abortion, sodomy, transgenderism, genocide, and the emergence of a full-fledged secularist, totalitarian technocracy), and it is easy to see we have truly transitioned into a physical, moral, intellectual, cultural, political, and spiritual Age of Unreality.

We know from Sacred Scripture and Tradition that a Great Tribulation will come upon the world during which the Antichrist will make his first personal appearance, coinciding with a great chastisement and persecution of Christians under his behest. After this, along with his counterfeit "church" now globally established and ubiquitous among Catholics and non-Catholics alike—"even the elect will be deceived, if that were possible"[1]—he will be vanquished, followed by an Era of Peace in which Christ in the Eucharist will reign over the world in a spiritual state of supernatural and natural harmony, a civilization of love. The Age of Unreality we are now in is, if not the complete establishment of this counterfeit global "church," the inauguration of it; and we are undoubtedly now living in the Great Tribulation.

Real Christian University (RCU)

In the remainder of this essay and in a follow-up essay, I would like to inquire into the kind of college or university that would need to be founded to educate young people most effectively in and for the Age of Unreality. I shall call this hypothetical institution, "Real Christian University" (RCU). My thesis is that such a university would have to be both radically traditional and radically innovative. The kind of teachers, students, curriculum, and pedagogy that enable any university's mission to succeed must be determined in light

---

[1] Matthew 24:24 (NIV)

of that mission; and the mission of any university must be determined in light of both the perennial and universal principles of education and the human soul and the exigencies and dictates of the time and place of its founding.

As a robustly Christian and integrally classical, liberal-arts university founded in early twenty-first century America, RCU would have only to consult as her models the successful colleges and universities of similar mission that have preceded her in the last several decades to discover these perennial principles in both theory (in their founding documents) and in practice (in the concrete and dynamic life and shape of their communities). Thus, RCU would take its essential core from the Christian, predominantly Catholic, intellectual, and educational tradition and institutional models that have recently been built upon it. But these institutions, however excellent and resonant with our mission, were founded before the Age of Unreality had reached and revealed the fullness of its nature. Thus, their capacity to serve as models for a similar institution founded in 2021 is significantly limited. The cultural and educational crises to which these colleges' founders responded were profound—the culture of death, secularism, scientism, the dictatorship of relativism, the instrumentalization and fragmentation of curriculum, the loss of wonder—but none of them compare to the crisis we now face, for it is both the synthesis and culmination of all of them: the global, totalitarian, technocratic supplanting of Reality by a man-made counterfeit.

Thus, in addition to being traditional and conservative, RCU would need to be radical and experimental. Józef Życiński has written:

To live the faith of Abraham is to be ready at a day's notice to pack the tents symbolizing everything that is dear to one and to go to a new, unknown place, which God will indicate, completely independently of rational calculations or our emotional predilections. To live the faith of Abraham in the cultural context of postmodernity is to be able calmly to pack up the tents of congenial concepts and arguments, not in order to set out on a desert path, but to set them up again in a different context and in a different form, in a place indicated by God. In an Abrahamic testimony of faith, one may not lose heart on account of the wildness of new places or on account of a feeling of loneliness in a foreign landscape. We must constantly seek the face of the Lord (Psalm 27:8), listening carefully to His voice, which could be either a discreet whisper or a delicate breeze (1 Kings 19:12). We need to love God more than the logic of convincing deductions and the collection of respected authorities, to which we like to refer in times of difficulty. We need to accept the provisionality of contingent means, in order that the Divine Absolute might all the more clearly reveal in them his power. Only then does the contemporary "wandering Aramaean" reveal the style in which, amidst the darkness of our doubt, flashes the light of the great adventure of our faith.[2]

---

[2] Józef Życiński, *God and Post-Modern Thought: Philosophical Issues in the Contemporary Critique of Modernity* Polish Philosophical Studies, IX, Translated by Kenneth W. Kemp and Zuzanna Maślanka Kieroń (Washington, D.C.: The Council for Research in Values and Philosophy, 2010), 130.

For our purposes, the "tents of congenial concepts and arguments" are the curricula of the predominantly and traditionally
Christian, integrated liberal-arts colleges and universities. The "different context" is the Age of Unreality. The "place indicated by God"
is yet to be determined. As for the "different form," we will attempt
to set this out in the remainder of this essay and in a future essay,
but we can say now that whatever form the "faith of Abraham" must
take for today, it will not only have to incorporate, integrate, and
transmit the classical and predominantly Catholic intellectual and
educational tradition, modeling itself upon them, but also render
this tradition fit and fruitful for an age whose discontinuity from all
preceding ones is all but absolute.

An Education into Reality

Many Catholic colleges and universities have articulated well the
perennial principles and curriculum of Catholic liberal education in
their founding documents. And their foundings share essentially the
same *raison d'etre*, though expressed differently according to their
particular charisms. The reality of American Catholic higher education to which their founding was a grace-ordained response was *etsi
Deus non daretur*, "as if God did not exist." Of course, there were
then courses offered in the humanities, philosophy, and theology
where the idea of God was discussed, but His reality was not taken
seriously by a critical mass of students, faculty, and administrators—
especially the large, big-name ones that I need not mention. If it had
been, the end result of four years at these institutions would have
been, and be, greater Faith, wisdom, and holiness in the graduates,

instead of greater confusion, immorality, worldliness, and apostasy. For the newer integrally Catholic colleges and universities, taking the reality of God seriously meant revising of the entire curriculum and culture to be ordered mainly to the study of God as its first principle and end, with the reality of God as the heart of their institutions' mission.

When the Living God, the Most Holy Trinity, was dethroned from Catholic higher education in America, reality itself became obscured. For God is ultimate reality, and when education leaves God aside through practical atheism, or relegates Him to one belief or idea among others through theological relativism and subjectivism, it is bound to become an education into the unreal, regardless of how 'scholarly' or 'scientific' it might claim to be. As Frank Sheed wrote decades ago:

> Therefore if we see anything at all—ourself or some other man, or the universe as a whole or any part of it—without at the same time seeing God holding it there, then we are seeing it all wrong. If we saw a coat hanging on a wall and did not realize that it was held there by a hook, we should not be living in the real world at all, but in some fantastic world of our own in which coats defied the law of gravity and hung on walls by their own power. Similarly if we see things in existence and do not in the same act see that they are held in existence by God, then equally we are living in a fantastic world, not the real world. Seeing God everywhere and all things upheld by Him is not a matter of sanctity, but of plain sanity, because God IS everywhere and all things are upheld

by Him. What we do about it may be sanctity; but merely seeing it is sanity. To overlook God's presence is not simply to be irreligious; it is a kind of insanity, like overlooking anything else that is actually there.[3]

For Sheed, education into reality meant first reauthorizing the Church in Catholic education, and not just one community of like-minded religious believers among others, but as the true and unique Mystical Body of Christ whose infallible teachings on nature, humanity, and God, and whose eternal-life-giving sacraments and liturgy serve as the bulwark and guide for all learning. And it meant a rejection of the anti-tradition of Enlightenment scientism, naturalism, and pragmatism, with its soulless curriculum of fractured disciplines ordered to will-to-power and ideology. It meant a return to the medieval, sapiential Tradition of the marriage of Faith and reason, with its soul-nourishing curriculum of the trivial and quadrivial arts and humanities ordered to the architectonic natural and divine sciences of philosophy and theology. The means of education are determined by its subject and end. The subject is the human person who is to be educated, and the end is the transformation we seek to make in his soul. The telos of this educational transformation is, generically, the same for all ages and places—perfection of the human soul and person through attainment of contemplative wisdom in intellectual virtue through perfecting of the speculative, or contemplative, powers of the intellectual soul and moral virtue through perfection of prudential powers of choice within the same soul.

---

[3] Frank Sheed, *Theology and Sanity* (San Francisco: Ignatius Press, 1947), 18.

In modern cultures, this end is prudentially adapted to the exigencies of practical life, including an orientation of the curriculum and pedagogy to the needs of the Church for evangelization and vocations, the common good of large-scale, technologically conditioned political and economic order, and the flourishing of family life through professional education and career success. This is not to say that liberal education must become mere job training and preparation for career, but only that it must have an eye to these things as at least indirect, subordinate, and prudent, or common sense, ends. The various curricula developed by these colleges were identical in the end to which they were ordered: natural and supernatural contemplative wisdom. Thus, they were also very similar in fundamental content and pedagogy, with philosophy, theology, and Great Books at the core, and Socratic discussion as the primary mode of teaching and learning. The trivial arts, mathematics and the natural sciences, and classical languages were also considered essential and given varied but serious weight, and lecture and pure seminar were employed, again, to varying extents, to complement the primary pedagogy of Socratic dialectic.

The main differences were in emphasis and charism, with colleges like Thomas More and the University of Dallas focusing more on humanities, Thomas Aquinas College giving Thomistic philosophy pride of place, and Wyoming Catholic College attempting a balanced synthesis of theology, philosophy, and humanities undergirded by an experiential outdoor curriculum ordered to physical, emotional, and moral virtue. All sought to provide their students a deep, comprehensive, and integrated immersion in the Real, both imaginatively, intellectually, and spiritually (with WCC including physically), through a curriculum and institutional milieu grounded in the Catholic intellectual, spiritual, and cultural tradition and leading their students from wonder to wisdom to God.

RCU would be no different from the aforementioned colleges and universities in being a Catholic and classical "school of reality," with its curriculum, pedagogy, and culture essentially modeled upon these institutions—there is no reason to reinvent the wheel. Yet, as all of these institutions were founded before the Age of Unreality, RCU could not use these as adequate models. Indeed, there is no model for her to use that would be adequate to her traditional, yet unprecedented mission. We are literally in unchartered territory. So, a sense exists in which the educational wheel must be reinvented. What would educational immersion in the Real look like in an Age of Unreality?

Lovers of the Real

The proper means of liberal education, especially the curriculum and pedagogy, is determined by the result at which it aims. Liberal education aims at the perfection of the rational powers of the soul of a rational animal—to the attainment of wisdom. To attain universal truth and be truly free, to contribute to the good of society, to engage in sound political activity based on a true understanding of the common good, and to articulate theological understanding and develop the habits necessary for the Christian life are the ends for which RCU would be established; and, in light of these ends, its curriculum and pedagogy would be essentially similar to the colleges that have come before it.

In all ages, the means to attain these perennial ends are also perennial: master teachers and master works in dialectical discussion, theology, philosophy, and the seven liberal arts in a community of learning ordered to truth and holiness. How these curricular and pedagogical means would themselves be applied to the educational end, the 'means to the means,' as it were, will be different, adapted to the particular language, culture, habits of mind, and exigences of the place and time in which they are engaged. For example, the medieval trivium and quadrivium have been radically revised and extended due to the exponential growth and complexity of the arts and sciences beginning in the Renaissance. And so, what a successful and fruitful liberal-arts college education means and requires for an eighteen-year-old, middle-class, homeschooled freshman in twenty-first century America is, however alike in essentials, dramatically different from what even a late-twentieth-century American student would have required, let alone a European or Middle Eastern one.

But in an Age of Unreality, the age-place-time requirements and hence the differences will need to be even more dramatic. For, again, what we are dealing with in our day is something unprecedented and unimaginable to prior generations. Therefore, RCU would teach theology according to the Catechism, the Encyclicals, Council Documents, the Fathers, and the Scholastics, as well as those modern and contemporary theologians faithful to the Deposit of the Faith. It would teach the perennial philosophy in accordance with the Catholic philosophical tradition, with St. Thomas Aquinas as master guide, again, along with those modern and contemporary philosophers who have continued and developed this tradition. And while it will teach the humanities, contemporary physical sciences, and the fine arts in an integrally Catholic manner ordered to the True, Good, and Beautiful, the exigencies of our time would require a radical and innovative adaption of these perennial sources and disciplines.

We must prepare future evangelists and religious for a Church that has been deeply coopted by the evilest of forces, and for a world that is awash in the most sophisticated, effective, and malicious propaganda ever created, causing the vast majority of people in the world to be in a perpetual state of psychological trauma and delusion. We must prepare future Catholic families to flourish in a world where men and women no longer exist as stable identities, where children are seen as exploitable commodities or insufferable burdens, and where marriage no longer exists as a natural, let alone a supernatural, reality. We cannot afford merely to have 'an eye' to these challenges. We must incorporate them intimately and intrinsically in the curriculum and pedagogy. This does not entail any essential change in the traditional Catholic liberal-arts program in its means and end but it does mean more than keeping these challenges in the background. RCU must face them head on.

We still need to delve into the details of what this would look like in terms of mission, curriculum, pedagogy, and culture. To give you a taste, let's just say that Jacques Ellul's *Propaganda*, Andrzej Łobaczewski's *Political Ponerology*, and the complete works of René Girard will be some of the Great Books we study; courses will include the liberal art of deconstructing media and government narratives, the history of false-flag terrorism, the nature of the Deep State, Catholic prophecies if Antichrist, and the reality and power of occult societies, such as Freemasonry. There will be practical, skills courses on economic independence and self-sufficiency. There will be deep teaching in psychology, especially psychopathy, narcissism, and ritual scapegoating. In sum, to claim that our students will become aware of the actual world in which they live and adept at Socratic inquiry and dialectics would be a bit of an understatement. Lastly, education of their hearts to love the One, Good, True, and Beautiful will take precedence over mere intellectual formation. For it is only wise and prudent, loving and courageous hearts that can supplant the Age of Unreality with the Civilization of Love, and usher in the Great Era of Peace.

Why Reading Plato is Necessary for Salvation—Now

In his *Confessions*,[4] St. Augustine remarked that he found all the fundamental truths in Plato... except the Incarnation. Well, that's a pretty big *except*. And if true, which it is—nowhere in the entire corpus of Plato is there even a hint of the "Good beyond Being" ever mixing itself with matter, for while the eternal and immutable forms may manifest themselves to us, they could, by metaphysical necessity, never descend to our world of time and space. If Augustine's remark is accurate, it would constitute a definitive answer to the question that is the title of this paper. For since the Incarnation of the Second Person of the Blessed Trinity *is* man's salvation; since the authoritative account of it is found nowhere else but in the Gospels; and since Plato, at least implicitly, denied its very possibility, then it would seem that in no way can reading Plato be necessary for salvation. Jesus Christ is *the* Way, the Truth, and the Life, and no one

---

4

comes to the Father except through Him; one must love the Lord with one's whole heart, mind, soul, and strength; love is impossible without knowledge of the beloved; and ignorance of Scripture, as St. Jerome said, is ignorance of Christ. Reading the Gospels, not Platonic dialogues, is what is necessary for salvation.

But even though we seem to have our answer, let's keep going. Let me share a brief story: In a weird time of my life, when I was working on my dissertation, I landed a job tutoring the children of a multi-millionaire traditionalist Catholic in Santa Cruz, California. I was charged with teaching all six of them, one-on-one, all of the liberal arts as well as theology. Well, one day I came to the house, and all the literature books in the library were replaced with Lives of the Saints. I asked the father of my students what had happened to the library, and he said something like, "Mr. Kozinski, I realized last night that all that matters is my children's salvation, that we are saved by being good Christians, and that the best Christians are the Saints, so they should be reading their lives—not Charles Dickens!"

Even though it is true that all that really matters is our salvation, there is something off with this mentality. But what is it precisely? Perhaps it has to do with the paradox that even though happiness is what we desire above all, if we try too hard to obtain happiness, concentrating on it alone as a goal, instead of just doing the things that we love and trying to God's will, we end up miserable. Perhaps it is the same with salvation—we must desire salvation, surely, but we attain it by desiring God for *His* own sake, more than for *our* salvation. Somehow revelation, faith, grace, the sacraments—though these are *necessary* for our salvation, they are not *sufficient*. But why not? To explore this question, and to see if indeed reading Plato is somehow necessary for salvation, we shall first describe what I would like to call "existential Platonism," which is more of a mindset and attitude than a set of philosophical doctrines. Then, we shall examine the culture we live in to show why existential Platonism is the natural antidote to its anti-*logos* immanentism and materialism. Next, we shall examine what Karl Rahner called "everyday mysticism," and discuss why this is the spiritual mode of being that God is calling us to, and why existential Platonism is its necessary complement and condition. Lastly, we shall discuss how Platonic dialectic as an intellectual ascesis or discipline can help up obtain "metaphysical courage," and avoid intellectual idolatry.

Existential Platonism

We have heard the story of Abraham Lincoln being educated on nothing but the Bible and Shakespeare. Prescinding from the exact truth of this narrative for a moment, why not just the Bible? Even if we say that of the two, the Bible is vastly more important for our souls, is not our intuition that the Bible cannot really be read profitably without Shakespeare, that is to say, without something like a liberal arts education, which, while not teaching us about the inner life of God and His dealings with human beings, allows us to understand human beings and the world to which the God of the Bible revealed Himself? How can we understand the Gospels if we do not have a deep and accurate understanding of the human nature that God subsumed into His Divinity, a human nature about which no one, except perhaps for Plato, wrote more profoundly, comprehensively, and accurately than Shakespeare? The liberal arts, the trivium and quadrivium, were considered, before modernity, indispensable tools for understanding the Bible. So, the liberal arts have some role in our salvation. But what about Plato?

We are born separated from God, and we are saved through grace, which makes us one again with the Divine, makes us children of God, and it is this reestablished kinship with God that constitutes our salvation. But before grace can render us children of God and divinize our souls, our souls must yearn for this sonship, this divinization. What makes us so yearn? A sense of the inadequacy and shadow-like nature of this world, an intense feeling of alienation and homesickness, and a profound intuition that there is much more to reality than what ordinarily appears to us. Plato's dialogues, I would argue, more than any other non-revealed writing man has ever penned, evoke these senses, feelings, and intuitions.

We know that Jesus Christ is *the answer* to the ultimate desires of the human heart. But what *about* the *question*? Can there really be an answer without a prior question? And can an answer be an answer for *me*, unless it is the answer to *my* question? Jesus Christ is our Salvation, but is He salvation for *me* unless I first *desire* this salvation? Eric Voegelin, the great twentieth-century German Platonist, wrote, "There is no answer to the Question other than the Mystery as it becomes luminous in the acts of questioning."[5] Paradoxically, then, the answers to spiritual questions are found in the questions themselves, or better, in the very act of questioning, the art of which was brought to perfection in practice by Plato's teacher Socrates, and in writing by Plato himself.

---

[5] Eric Voegelin, *The Ecumenic Age* (University of Missouri Press, 1974), 414.

Along with how to inquire into Being, Plato teaches us the essential spiritual and metaphysical truths, as well as the mystical habit of mind and soul, without which Faith and Grace are stillborn in our souls. We must believe in the biblical God through obedience to revelation, but do we not need to some extent *know* that He exists, and know it intimately and existentially? If we believe by Faith and even know by experience that He exists, but we cannot reconcile the revealed doctrine of His providential care of all material things with what our modernized, materialized, mechanized, and Darwinized minds tell us, then we are part atheist in our souls. If we believe by Faith that He cares for us, but everything in us *but* our Faith tends to see human power in perpetual battle with inexorable chaos, then we suffer from a dividedness of soul that is spiritually perilous. If our Faith tells us that absolute Goodness exists, but our souls cannot see anything absolute in a world that has been flatted, demythologized, and disenchanted through the imposition of an immanent frame, then we are in danger of believing with one divinely infused part of us, and disbelieving with all the other natural powers. We are told in the Scriptures and the Church that we have an eternal soul, but can we be truly faithful to a truth that is alien to our everyday awareness and intellectual paradigms? God is spirit, we are told by the Church, and so we must believe that there is more to reality than matter, but compared to the men of the ancient and medieval worlds, we tend towards an unconscious materialism.

Plato can teach us to see "the world in a grain of sand" and "eternity in an hour" as the great mystic and Platonist William Blake wrote. He can teach us to see the absolute through the relative, the immutable in the mutable, the divine in the profane. It is Plato above all who teaches us those natural truths dispositive to the fruitful reception of revelation: the existence of the Absolute Good, His providential interest and care for the world, the existence and immortality of the soul, the symbolically charged character of all material things. We cannot be saved, or it will be much harder than it has to be if we do not *experience* these realities, even if we ultimately accept them in obedience to Divine Faith.

In short, in Plato's capacity to prompt recognition of our alienation from truth, to provide us a mystical glimpse of this true reality, to evoke a perpetual yearning for it, and enable us, through the dialectical method of inquiry he invented, to achieve some participation in it by a diligent ascesis of mind, he is simply indispensable, both as a precursor to Faith, and a guide along the way to our heavenly home. Max Scheler, the great twentieth-century German phenomenologist and sociologist, captures well the existential Platonism I have been recommending:

This new attitude might first of all be characterized vaguely enough from the emotional point of view as a surrender of self to the intuitional content of things, as a movement of profound trust in the unshakableness of all that is simply given, as a courageous letting oneself-go in intuition and in the loving movement toward the world in its capacity for being intuited. This philosophy faces the world with the outstretched gesture of the open hand and the wide-eyed gaze of wonder. This is not the squinting, critical gaze that Descartes—beginning with the universal doubt—casts upon things, nor the eye of Kant, from which comes a spiritual beam so alien as, in its dominating fashion, it penetrates the world of things. The man who philosophizes with the new attitude has neither the anxiety characteristic of modem calculation and the modem desire to verify things, nor the proud sovereignty of the "thinking reed which in Descartes and Kant is the original source—the emotional a priori of all their theories. Instead, the stream of being flows in on him, and seeps down to his spiritual roots, as a self-evident benevolent element, simply that, apart from all content. This surrender to being is characterized by love, a willingness to be dominated rather than to dominate, to bathe in the richness of being rather than to impoverish being by seeking to control it for the sake of one's own subjective assurance.[6]

Faith, by which we are saved, is not reducible to the affirmation of doctrinal propositions, for it is the substance of things hoped for, the evidence of things unseen. We need an existential encounter with the God who transcends subjectivity and human consciousness, but, nevertheless, can be touched by us, as von Balthasar puts it: "Suddenly and in an indescribable manner the ray of the Unconditional breaks through, casting a person down to adoration and transforming him into a believer and a follower."[7] It is meeting the living God in the depths of our souls, not merely adhering stubbornly to beliefs about Him, that saves us. Jesus said that unless you

---

[6] Max Scheler, *Trust of People, Words, and God: A Route for Philosophy of Religion* (University of Notre Dame Press, 1980), 19.

[7] Hans Urs von Balthasar, *The Glory of the Lord: A Theological Aesthetic, Volume I: Seeing the Form* (Ignatius Press, 1982), 33.

become a little child, you cannot enter the Kingdom of God. What I am calling "existential Platonism," is, I think, tantamount to the natural spiritual childlikeness of which Our Lord speaks.

The Enemies of Logos

A flower cannot grow in infertile soil, may even die, or not even be born in the first place. Our present culture is, among all the myriad descriptions one could give it, anti-*logos*, rather than simply anti-Christian. Listen to Hans Urs Von Balthasar describe the Western world in the 1960s, a world in which the enemies of *Logos* were only just beginning their all-out onslaught.

> In a world without beauty—even if people cannot dispense with the word and constantly have it on the tip of their tongues in order to abuse it—in a world which is perhaps not wholly without beauty, but which can no longer see it or reckon with it: In such a world the good also loses its attractiveness, the self-evidence of why it must be carried out. Man stands before the good and asks himself why it must be done and not rather its alternative, evil. For this, too, is a possibility, and even the more exciting one: Why not investigate Satan's depths? In a world that no longer has enough confidence in itself to affirm the beautiful, the proofs of the truth have lost their cogency. In other words, syllogisms may still dutifully clatter away like rotary presses or computers which infallibly spew out an exact number of answers by the minute. But the logic of these answers is itself a mechanism

which no longer captivates anyone. The very conclusions are no longer conclusive. And if this is how the transcendentals fare because one of them has been banished, what will happen with Being itself?[8]

Thus, we need existential Platonism more than any other post-Christian age did, for Platonism at its core aims at the visceral experience of *logos*, of order, of an enchanted, soaring, mystical reason that touches the real true, good, and beautiful, of the absolute and transcendent in the thick of the contingent and immanent, of the divine in everything and at every moment. Josef Pieper wrote, in his great commentary on Plato's *Phaedrus*:

> For the general public is being reduced to a state where people not only are unable to find about the truth but also become unable to search for the truth because they are satisfied with deception and trickery that have determined their convictions, satisfied with a fictitious reality created by design through the abuse of language.[9]

Plato singlehandedly took the sorely abused language of his Athens and lovingly rehabilitated it to become the primary conduit for the human translation of the Divine *Logos* which came to us four centuries later. We need Plato's help now to do the same for the tortured and mutilated discourse of our day. Alasdair MacIntyre:

---

[8] Ibid., 18.

[9] Josef Pieper, *Abuse of Language – Abuse of Power* (Ignatius Press, 1992), 47.

229 Chapter IV: Apocalypse

We have within our social order few if any social milieus within which reflective and critical enquiry concerning the central issues of human life can be sustained.... This tends to be a culture of answers, not of questions, and those answers, whether secular or religious, liberal or conservative, are generally delivered as though meant to put an end to questioning.[10]

The death of questioning, of inquiry, of what Eric Voegelin called "existential unrest," is the death of the soul. Thus, ours is a culture of not just physical but spiritual death. The life blood of man's soul is spiritual and existential inquiry—"Why?" Why? Why? The child asks, and when he loses his innocence he ceases to do so, or only out of self-serving curiosity, for he has become self-sufficient, impervious to a sense of the mystery of Being, whether he is a faithful believer in God or not. Insofar as the ideology and spirit of secularism and liberalism, technocratism, anthropocentric humanism, mammonism, and moral relativism incarnate itself every deeper into everyday life, the existence of a reality other than naked human will and desire and its various artifacts becomes less and less apparent and available to the soul. Charles Taylor calls this trajectory the Immanent Frame. And not only is the supernatural banished from consciousness, but the natural as well. Romano Guardini tells us that we live "at the end of the modern world," modernity being the apotheosis of the trinity of nature, culture, and man, and post-modernity its rejection in an unnatural nature, anti-cultural

---

[10] Alasdair MacIntyre, *After Virtue* (University of Notre Dame Press, 1981), 263.

culture, and inhuman man. The upshot of all this is that we are living in the first culture whose primary habituating effect is to render repentance, and thus salvation, as close to impossible as possible. Peter Kreeft:

> C.S. Lewis says, in "The Poison of Subjectivism," that relativism "will certainly end our species and damn our souls." Why does he say "damn our souls?" Because Lewis is a Christian, and he does not disagree with the fundamental teaching of his master, Christ, and all the prophets in the Jewish tradition, that salvation presupposes repentance, and repentance presupposes an objectively real moral law. Moral relativism eliminates that law, thus trivializes repentance, thus imperils salvation.[11]

If Plato teaches us anything, and if reading Plato has any effect on our souls, it is this: The Good exists, and we are not it; it is absolute, demands our obedience, is thoroughly knowable by every human being; finally, that it is in searching for, knowing, and obeying this Good, which we can encounter in the very heart of our souls, that we are become happy, and are rendered pure so as to possess this happiness forever. We need to repent to be saved, but we need first to believe in and encounter the Good in the created world before we can meet Him in the Creator.

---

[11] Peter Kreeft, *A Refutation of Moral Relativism: Interviews with an Absolutist* (Ignatius Press, 1999), 47.

Everyday Mysticism

I now want to try to describe the mode of spiritual consciousness and practice I think God is calling us to, and why an existential Platonism of the heart is the best preparation for these graces. I believe that Romano Guardini's depiction of the future that he penned in 1956 is true, and I believe the future he envisioned is now. He wrote:

> The new age will declare that the secularized facets of Christianity are sentimentalities. This declaration will clear the air. The world to come will be filled with animosity and danger, but it will be a world open and clean.... As unbelievers deny Revelation more decisively, as they put their denial into more consistent practice, it will become the more evident what it really means to be a Christian. At the same time, the unbeliever will emerge from the fogs of secularism. He will cease to reap benefit from the values and forces developed by the very Revelation he denies. He must learn to exist honestly without Christ and without the God revealed through Him; he will have to learn to experience what this honesty means. Nietzsche has already warned us that the non-Christian of the modern world had no realization of what it truly meant to be without Christ. The last decades have suggested what life without Christ really is. The last decades were only the beginning.[12]

---

[12] Romano Guardini, *The End of the Modern World* (San Francisco: Ignatius Press, 1956), 123.

Guardini does not leave us without hope, or a practical prescription for action in this frightening apocalyptic scenario. He tells us that "free union of the human person with the Absolute through unconditional freedom will enable the faithful to stand firm—God—centered—even though placeless and unprotected." "Loneliness in faith will be terrible. Love will disappear from the face of the public world, but the more precious will be that love that flows from one lonely person to another, involving a courage of the heart born from the immediacy of the love of God as it was made known in Christ.... Perhaps love will achieve an intimacy and harmony never known to this day."[13]

This immediacy of the love of God, and this harmonious and courageous and intimate love for our neighbor, seem to indicate a new and higher mode of Christian spirituality, what one might call an *existential* Christianity. This does not mean that a dogmatic, ecclesial, sacramental, liturgical, charismatic Christianity is thereby excluded or even deemphasized. It just means, I think, that absent a deep existential component, without a mystical intimacy with and awareness of the living God in our hearts, we will not be able to withstand the onslaught of the anti-logos nihilism and lovelessness that awaits us. What Guardini is describing is an experience of God that goes beyond images and concepts. Raimon Panikkar puts it profoundly: "The touch with the real without the mediation of consciousness is precisely the mystical."[14] I think Panikkar here sums up

---

[13] Ibid, 86.

[14] Raimon Panikkar, *The Rhythm of Being: The Gifford Lectures* (Orbis Books, 2009), 247.

the deeper teaching of Plato, who was trying to tell us in his dialogues that all words, images, and thoughts are merely fingers pointing at the Sun, but never the Sun itself, and that it is precisely in recognizing the limitations of human thought and consciousness that the Sun, the Good beyond Being, can be touched, or rather, can touch us. Yes, we need to go to Mass and confession (if we are Catholics), to keep to a discipline of prayer, virtue, and good works, to study Christian doctrine, to "keep the Faith." But are we merely going through the motions? What did Our Lord mean when he said, "Not everyone who says to Me, "Lord, Lord," shall enter the kingdom of heaven, but he who does the will of My Father in heaven"? If the emotional, psychological, and spiritual comfort and security of our Benedict Option fortresses is making these kinds of radical acts of love, obedience, and abandonment to the will of God nonexistent, or just rare, then maybe we should depart from them, or even destroy them.

Plato teaches us that every particular being we experience is always and already more than itself, for each bespeaks a transcendent and mysterious fullness of being of which it is a partial constituent as well as a mystical pointer. But the deepest teaching of Plato is that reality not only exceeds the written word, as the *Phaedrus* teaches, but also the spoken word. For, ultimate reality exceeds thought and consciousness altogether—yet we can still somehow touch it, or allow it to touch us. This is what arising out of the cave and ascending the ladder of love to the top of the divided line amount to—the experience of the Real beyond thought, even beyond consciousness. St. Paul wrote, "For the invisible things of him since the creation of the world, are clearly seen, being perceived through the things that are made."[15] We have all but lost this Platonic vision, and the fructification of grace in our souls requires its recovery.

Metaphysical Courage: To Infinity and Beyond

Over three hundred years ago, Blaise Pascal decried the state of his society: "Truth is so obscured nowadays and lies so well established, that unless we love the truth we shall never see it."[16] Pascal's description of his day is a fortiori descriptive of ours, as purpose, meaning, coherence, order, and love, things that make existence endurable and enjoyable, are diminishing fast as a function of our collective cowardice. It is not that truth is not available in our society, but that its being found is a function of our desire for it—and we lack this desire, for we have lost hope in the Truth. As our pluralistic society falls into pieces and becomes ever more fractured into disparate groups with irreconcilable worldviews, the need for a uniting intellectual and moral consensus becomes more and more urgent, and this can only be one centered in *Logos*. But because radically different worldviews have radically different first principles, it is very difficult to come to an agreement on the existence and nature of this Logos through argument alone; and since each group has its own unique philosophical starting point and mode of discourse, argument, discussion, and debate are becoming more and more futile.

---

[15] Romans 1:20 (King James Version).

[16] Blaise Pascal, *Pensées*, trans. A.J. Krailsheimer (Penguin Classics, 1995), 123.

We all need—traditional Christians not excluded—to question boldly our assumptions and reflect rigorously upon our first principles. Do we have a courageous understanding of what is real, or do we hide fearfully in false first premises and partial truths we take to be the whole? Are we open to correction, because we see that our consciousnesses always, to some extent, distort reality? Are we truly open to the deepest truth of reality, that it is wild, unsafe, ultimately exceeds our grasp and control, but, is, nevertheless, good and trustworthy? Or do we prefer the secure mental order we create for ourselves? If a lack of mental manhood is the underlying cause of our cultural decline, then we need to take mental risks and perform feats of spiritual endurance in the midst of overwhelming odds. But with the extrinsic help of Tradition, the intrinsic help of grace, and our cooperation with this grace through courageous and relentless inquiry and dialogue in the Platonically existential mode, coupled with our practice of everyday mystical contemplation, we can ascend now, at least partially, to the whole which awaits us personally in the Beatific Vision.

Well, we have yet to hear from Plato, so he can have the last word:

When a man is always occupied with the cravings of desire and ambition, and is eagerly striving to satisfy them, all his thoughts must be mortal, and, as far as it is possible altogether to become such, he must be mortal every whit, because he has cherished his mortal part. But he who has been earnest in the love of knowledge and of true wisdom, and has exercised his intellect more than any other part of him, must have thoughts immortal and divine, if he attain truth, and in so far as human nature is capable of sharing in immortality, he must altogether be immortal; and since he is ever cherishing the divine power, and has the divinity within him in perfect order, he will be perfectly happy.[17]

I will put in place salvation for he who longs for it: A Meditation on Psalm 12

Psalm 12 speaks to us today, right now. The Psalmist cries out for protection and salvation from the deceptive, idolatrous, and lawless, as the poor are devastated and groaning in agony, and the lover and speaker of Truth is banished and excluded. The Lord hears the cry and responds. His response was the same then as it is now and will be in the future, as the devastation and groaning rise to insufferable levels, and the banished and excluded are violently persecuted and murdered. It is not the response we may want, but the one we need.

"Truly the Covenant Lover has ceased to have a place; truly the truthful-faithful do not appear among the sons of men." This describes the present state of the world perfectly, but its understated expression conceals untold horror. The City of God, the remnant of those who still love and obey truth, is eclipsed, gone, lost, unpresent. Only the City of Man remains. Thus, the world that we see and experience and live within, a world that we are being *made* to see, experience, and live within through psychological and spiritual manipulation of the most sophisticated and totalitarian kind, is bereft

---

[17] Plato, *Timaeus*, trans. Donald J. Zeyl (Dover Publications, 2008), 49.

of being, of reality, of love, of truth, of God. It is a hell on earth that is emerging, and is all but here. The plandemic was the perfect instantiation of this, where those who spoke the truth, and the truths they spoke, were disappeared from existence. Only the Covenant Hater and the mendacious and treacherous had a place and appeared among the sons of men, including the sons of the Church, who were among the most mendacious and treacherous. In the Church now the few orthodox and repentant left among the clergy and laity have lost all public authority and influence, and are forced to hide together in virtual catacombs and upper rooms, both for fear of the Jews—saying "Christ is King" is now "antisemitic"—and for fear of the "Catholics," those who follow the Usurper.

"These speak deceptively, each man to his neighbor, with idolatrous lips in the heart. And thus their heart speaks!"

Lies are the lingua franca of today's City of Man, and idolatry is its only commerce. And these are both the cause and the effect of the public disappearance of the faithful. Notice that the Psalmist places these together, as they must be. For a lie is always an idol, and an idol is always a lie. As Josef Pieper teaches us, our words remove a piece of reality from the person to whom we lie, for words reveal and transmit reality, and lies are anti-words eclipsing and occluding reality. And since the greatest reality is God, the act of idolatry in speech is the greatest lie, removing God from human discourse by replacing Him with words signifying nothing. From our hearts come words that either speak God into existence for ourselves and others, in imitation of the Sacred Heart of the Word Incarnate, or they speak Him out of existence through idolatrous deception. Every word authorized to appear in the public square, which itself is a virtual simulacrum of reality, speaks God out of existence, and any unauthorized, godly ones that happen to get through are immediately twisted into their opposite or just directed to the nearest memory hole, which are ubiquitous. A man is a woman. Mutilation is care. A bioweapon is a vaccine. A same-sex couple being blessed is not blessing a *same-sex* couple. Genocide is self-defense. We never said the vaccine was safe and effective. Food and housing were never cheaper in the past, and the cities are cleaner and safer than they have ever been. Totalitarianism is a thing of the past.

"May the LORD cut off all idolatrous lips, the tongue that utters great words, those who say, 'By our tongue we are mighty; our lips are our own, who is lord to us?'" The Psalmist has presented the reader with the problem in his day, as it is in ours, and he requests from God an apt solution. The problem is that his world was dominated by those who made themselves God, for they rejected all authority other than power, and their own power at that. And they attained this domination by lying. The global totalitarianism that is now almost complete, perhaps to be ushered in *in tota* by the next and final scamdemic presided over by Antichrist and his minions in Church and Empire, was nothing but the systematic, technocratic, bureaucratic installation of lies, with the complicity of many of the lied-to, a situation described to perfection by George Orwell in *1984*. Since God has all the power, the solution is for God to destroy the idols and disempower their ability to lie. Notice that the Psalmist doesn't demand that they themselves be destroyed, only their power to sin, or at least the effects of it. This is a foreshadowing of the "Wheat and Tares" parable, as well as Our Lord's command to love our enemies. It is the perfect solution, it would seem, but God has another one, and for a different problem.

"Because of the devastation of the poor, of the groaning of the needy, now I arise," says the LORD. I will put in place salvation for he who longs for it." It is not because of the displacement of the righteous from public view and authority that God arises, but because of the suffering of the poor. It is the poor, those who always suffer the most from traitorous leaders when authority becomes pure power, who are helpless to defend themselves, and whose suffering goes most unnoticed and least cared about, for which God arises. But His solution is not to empower them materially or socially or to disempower their torturers. And it is not directed only at the poor, but also to the displaced righteous. And here we come to the most profound verse of the Psalm. God arises to "put in place salvation for he who longs for it."

Here we see most where this Psalm speaks to us, both the poor and the displaced righteous (well, repentant at best, and then only sometimes). I can't count the times I have asked God, especially since March of 2020, to arise and destroy all the evil (and not just by cutting off idolatrous lips . . .) He hasn't. And the evil keeps growing and becoming more intolerable, unspeakable, unfathomable. But for God, there is an even greater evil, the greatest evil, opposing the greatest good, the Evil for which He arises and always arises to destroy so that He may give us the good He wants us to have above all and always wants to give us. During these past few years I have tried to understand why God is allowing this level and extent of evil, a literal hell on earth, and what kept coming to me is this: It is to force us to cry out to Him. And this Psalm verse confirms this. The greatest good man can obtain is salvation, eternal life with God in Heaven, and the *sine qua non* of obtaining it is to desire it, to *long* for it. When we do this, God arises to give it to us. The greatest evil is eternal damnation, and what causes us to obtain it is also desire. When we do not desire salvation, when we long for lying idols instead, we are telling God that we do not want it, which is to say, that we would rather have damnation.

God will eventually cut off all idolatrous lips; indeed, he will annihilate the City of Man and the Antichrist, as the Book of Revelation tells us. And this will usher in the City of God on earth for "a thousand years." This is the Era of Peace, preceding the final onslaught of Antichrist and the End of Time. Perhaps we will live to see this Era, for the Great Chastisement that must precede is imminent, if not already upon us. And He will arise today, and is already doing so, but not by violent retribution for the evildoers and vindication of the just. This is just not happening, and will not happen until the End of the Era. What He *is* doing—and permitting—is everything He can to make us long for salvation, and He is putting salvation in place for those who do. Yes, we must denounce evil and stand up for the truth (and I wouldn't mind seeing all the plandemic villains, child mutilators, and Zionist mass murderers of Gazan women and children given the death penalty). But let us transform our great suffering and those of others into pangs of longing for God, for Heaven, for the Kingdom of His Divine Will.

"The words of the LORD are words without alloy, silver refined in a furnace on the earth, seven times purified. YOU, LORD, keep them with care, protect us forever from this generation. The lawless prowl all around, seeking exaltation, worthlessness is the lot of the sons of men." The words of the Lord—silver, not gold here, because incarnate and active and enmeshed in this debased world—are the antidote. He will keep us in His care, and protect us forever from this generation of the lawless as well as the Lawless One who is to come, soon. But His care is primarily for our souls, and He wants above all for us to long and increase our longing for His salvation, to become the Sons of God that we already are. This is our prime directive. Anything else compared to this is as worthless as the lot of the sons of men.

About the Author

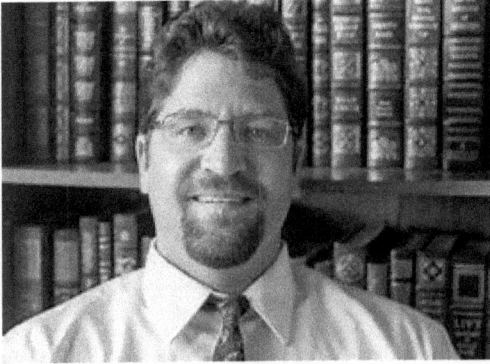

Dr. Thaddeus Kozinski is an advocate of Catholic liberal education and the Socratic method of teaching, and has authored a number of articles and books, including *The Political Problem of Religious Pluralism: And Why Philosophers Cannot Solve It* and *Modernity as Apocalypse: Sacred Nihilism and the Counterfeits of Logos*. He developed and taught a course on Reason in the Theology of St. Thomas at Holy Apostles College & Seminary in Cromwell, CT. At present, he teaches philosophy for Memoria College and John Adams Academy. He is the author of *Modernity as Apocalypse: Sacred Nihilism and the Counterfeits of Logos* (Angelico Press) and *Words, Concepts, Reality: Aristotelian Logic for Teenagers* (En Route).

www.ingramcontent.com/pod-product-compliance
Lightning Source LLC
Chambersburg PA
CBHW070027100426
42740CB00013B/2618